BODY OF KNOWLEDGE

THE COMPLETE
WEIGHT MANAGEMENT SYSTEM
FOR A LIFETIME OF HEALTH

DR. ROBERT J. MOORE III

Bridgeway
Books

BODY OF KNOWLEDGE: THE COMPLETE WEIGHT MANAGEMENT SYSTEM
FOR A LIFETIME OF HEALTH
PUBLISHED BY BRIDGEWAY BOOKS
P.O. BOX 80107
AUSTIN, TEXAS 78758

For more information about our books, please write to us, call
512.478.2028, or visit our web site at www.bridgewaybooks.net.

ISBN-13: 978-1-934454-08-4
ISBN-10: 1-934454-08-7

Library of Congress Control Number: 2007939728

10 9 8 7 6 5 4 3 2 1

I dedicate this book to all families.
To my daughters, Jessica and Samantha, for their unwavering
patience, understanding, and participation in this project.
To my parents and sister Cynthia, thank you for your continued
support, love, and gift of tenacity.

TABLE OF CONTENTS

ACKNOWLEDGMENTS

I would like to thank everyone who has kept this project as well as my vision and dream alive. There were many times when the book had to be shelved and when BOKsystems development came to a halt, but my science and business teams have always been there to support me and this project. The exalted feeling I have after finishing this book is overshadowed by the relationships and friendships I have made during the last ten years.

Because this book project was a huge undertaking, and the fact that I am sure I will be adding more people to the BOK family, I have placed the individual names on the web site. I am grateful to everyone we have encountered who has helped with this project and grateful to everyone who continues to address the present obesity and health care crises.

INTRODUCTION

A Personal Message:

Most doctors share a common dream—to help cure those who are in need and to do something really special in their career. While I enjoy every facet of my surgical practice, overall my professional sense of accomplishment has come from successfully helping people transform their lives through the Body of Knowledge™ system.

Body of Knowledge, or BOK™ (pronounced "Be Okay"), is the result of twenty years of study, research, and working with people who have come to me overweight, out of shape, and often despondent. I believe that my vision and expertise mirrors an emerging public demand for healthy lifestyle programs. I have found that most people prefer a blend of truth and essential information in an organized, facts-driven format over the gimmick-driven and "quick fix" weight loss plans of the past. This new enthusiasm could not have come at a better time. Serious health problems associated with weight gain in both adults and children are increasing across the nation. Even though there are more diet and fitness plans on the market than any time in history, there are more people considered obese and overweight than ever before (over half of our population). And I have special concern about the childhood obesity epidemic.

My quest is to help you design your own weight, fitness, and life-management plan; I'll give you the essential information and techniques you'll need to customize it to match your personal goals and lifestyle.

My personal message to you is this: there is no one better qualified to create a health plan for you than *you*. Use the Body of Knowledge system as your guide and consider me your teacher. My wish is for you to be armed with all the knowledge you need to once again take control of your health.

The BOKsystem is not a magic bullet or a fad diet but a sensible, sustainable program for managing weight and promoting good health. As you will see in the coming pages, the BOKsystem is designed to help individuals learn how a healthy body should function and how to "unlearn" their unhealthy habits. Then we use the BOKsystem to help individuals create a personal plan for healthy living that makes sense for them.

Body of Knowledge is also addressing the critical rise in health care costs. It is no coincidence that medical expenses and health insurance premiums mirror the rise in obesity cases and other related health problems. However, recent studies show that some overweight and obese employees who lost weight not only reduced their employers' health care costs but were also rewarded a portion of the savings, which encouraged them to keep the weight off longer. Better health results in proven savings for everyone. Individuals pay for fewer doctor visits, emergency room admissions, surgeries, and prescriptions. Companies save on a decrease in sick leave, fewer employees retrained, and reduced disability costs; they also benefit from the increase in productivity, innovation, and employee morale. In addition, allowing primary care physicians and specialists to utilize a more effective preventative care model instead of continuing to treat the end-stage diseases associated with obesity (heart disease, stroke, diabetes, cancer, etc.) is a win-win situation.

The Body of Knowledge system is exciting because it offers a realistic plan to help people make life-altering, life-affirming changes. If enough people take the precepts of Body of Knowledge to heart, it could have an impact beyond all of our dreams.

THE BOK MISSION

Our mission is to provide information that gives you the ability to create and maintain a healthy lifestyle that adapts to change—one that naturally manages your weight, keeps you fit, promotes good health, and gives you a Body of Knowledge.

What if we lived in a world where

- all food choices were healthy choices—made cost-effective and available due to consumer demand;
- fast food and junk food in the home, schools, and the workplace were eliminated;
- businesses and health insurance companies offered bonuses or incentives to reward employees and clients who achieve and maintain better health;
- parents and schools taught children the foundation of healthy living so no one was programmed with bad habits that follow them through life;
- obesity and health-related problems were only read about in history books.

This is my dream, my quest—to make sure that you and your family will B-OK. And I'll take it one meal, one workout, and one person at a time.

Good health and all my best,

Dr. B.

How to Use This Book

I developed the Body of Knowledge system to help people create a personalized fitness program that can adapt to their individual lifestyle. In the beginning, I encourage you to use this book as a reference guide. Make notes in the margins, tab important sections with color-coded flags, or do whatever suits your style. Recording details about the program and how it is affecting you will give you the ability to refer back to your notes later to see what gave you good, mediocre, or bad results. If you prefer to keep a daily or weekly written record, you can print your BOK Journal pages from the web site as you need them.

There's so much information about our bodies and health, it was necessary to move some of the book's content to the web so you wouldn't end up with a five hundred page tome! I also didn't want to limit this learning process to just ink and paper. With all the options the Internet offers, I hope to give you the opportunity to learn as much as you want and do it on your time schedule. The web site will allow you to find more details on interesting subjects from the book, see in-depth graphics and analyses, and *link* to other web sites that offer useful information. I hope you'll take advantage of this opportunity and not limit your learning to just what's contained in this book. Using the BOK web site to complement your reading will truly enhance your plan for total health and fitness.

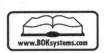

Web Icon: This icon will pop up often in the book, and it's your signal that more information on the subject you've been reading about is on the BOK web site. When you go to www.BOKsystems.com, you'll see this icon on the homepage. Click on it and you'll be directed to a listing of all the places this icon appears in the book, organized according to the five main parts and then by page number. Find the corresponding page number, click, and you'll have access to new information, graphics, charts, audio summaries, and more.

Audio Icon: This icon is located exclusively on the web site where you can hear a simplified version of a complicated subject that I have narrated for your convenience.

To give you an idea of what you're about to get into, I've put together a quick overview of the book:

PART 1 – WELCOME TO THE MACHINE: Before we get started on building a better you, you'll first need to understand what you are up against and learn how fad diets, super-sized food portions, and extreme exercise plans have conspired to undo your healthy you. In this section I will teach you the basics of how your machine works and help you gain the knowledge, motivation, and inspiration to get your personal machine back in tune with the world around you.

PART 2 – FOOD AND EATING HABITS: In this section I am going to help you rethink how, what, and why you eat. Somewhere along the line eating became a recreational hobby rather than a simple act of human survival. We'll untwist our "eating for fun" thinking and get back to the reality of eating for peak performance and health.

PART 3 – ACTIVITY AND EXERCISE: I think exercise should be as enjoyable as possible, and I hope by the end of this section you will too. At any age and fitness level I encourage you to rethink activity and exercise in terms of fun and relaxation. In fact, the right kind of exercise will make you feel good, which will make you want to exercise more—a healthy cycle that maintains itself. Together we'll design a fitness plan that's just right for you.

PART 4 – PUTTING IT ALL TOGETHER: By this point you'll be ready to take your newfound knowledge and put it all together. Design your own eating and exercise program from scratch or you can choose from the five BOK programs already designed for you and then modify them to fit your own preferences and needs on the BOK web site. The BOKsystem is a *complete* weight-management system, so we offer plans for healthy weight loss, weight maintenance, and even weight gain.

PART 5 – MIND OVER MATTER: Now that you'll know how and why good eating habits and a sensible exercise program can put you on the fast track to healthy living, I'll show you how avoid or navigate through the obstacles that keep you from reaching your goals. Your mind is the most powerful organ in your body, but you have to learn how it affects your body and use this knowledge to remove its unhealthy influences and avoid potential setbacks. Your Body of Knowledge program will be complete once you learn how to turn your thoughts and decisions into the healthy actions and results you want.

As you go through the book don't be afraid to skip around to different parts when you need some refreshing or a little extra inspiration. Revisiting concepts after you've read the entire book can really put things in a new light or change the way you plan to design your own BOK program. Now, enjoy yourself and have fun as you discover new facts, dispel old myths, and begin your journey toward your new Body of Knowledge.

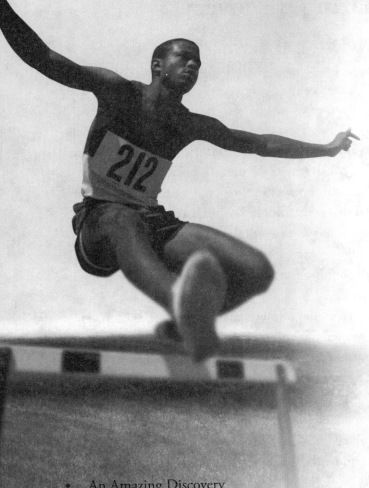

PART 1

WELCOME TO THE MACHINE

1

An Amazing Discovery

Today, many people know the sad statistics behind popular diets. About 90 to 95 percent of people in this country who lose weight gain some or all of it back within two years. This statistic has remained consistent since dieting became a focus in our society. Ironically, health problems associated with weight gain and obesity in both adults and children are increasing, while the diet and fitness industry continues to grow. Every day there is a new magic diet plan, pill, or exercise machine introduced to a willing audience of people looking for a quick fix. Clearly, we haven't gotten it right yet.

There are many factors in our lives that influence weight management, our health, or even our ability to make informed decisions, and the dominant gimmick-driven, quick-fix weight loss plans only address a handful of those factors. The good news is that there has been a backlash to the magic pill pursuit that has resulted in a very positive trend. People are finally seeking truthful, fact-driven information that will help them make educated decisions about their health. I will provide this information and teach you how to get better results and keep them for life.

MAKE THE MOST OF YOUR BOK EXPERIENCE

1. Visit the web site any time you see a 📖 icon to get more in-depth information, extra graphics, audio summaries, and more.
2. Make notes in the book margins and mark pages you want to continuously refer to.
3. Keep a journal or enter information in a day planner. You can go to the web site and print BOK Journal pages as you need them.
4. Make time to become familiar with the web site and its tools. It is your most complete source for daily information, record keeping, and motivation.
5. Skip around to the different parts of the book when you need some refreshing or a little extra inspiration.
6. Through continued reinforcement from the book and web site, you will master the BOK experience and learn how to attain a lifetime of health and fitness.

It has been proven that people who are able to lose weight and then manage it for life share some common truths. First, they have a sense of *autonomy*. They trust their own judgment, make good decisions, and have learned some good personal habits. Second, they do not consistently connect emotional highs and lows with food, but treat food as fuel to run their machine and promote good health. They've learned that the secret to losing weight and keeping it off is not just about calorie restriction but knowing what they are eating, when to eat it, and why they are eating it. Third, they have found a

> PEOPLE WHO ARE ABLE TO LOSE WEIGHT AND THEN MANAGE IT FOR LIFE ... HAVE A SENSE OF AUTONOMY.

way to make exercise simple, effective, and fun. As with everything else in life, knowledge is power, and you alone are ultimately responsible for your own health. The Body of Knowledge system is designed for one purpose and with one goal in mind—to provide you with the information and tools you need to maintain a healthy weight, to stay fit, and remain energetic for life! Before we get started, I want to share my own story with you.

The Medical Sleuth

A strange thing happened to me on the way to becoming a doctor. I discovered the secret to permanent weight loss and fitness.

It all started in the mid-1980s when I began studying for the Medical College Admission Test (MCAT). When I made the decision to take the test, I knew my life would change dramatically. Prior to this turning point, most of my life had revolved around organized sports. By my sophomore year in college, reality took hold. I stopped playing football (though I still worked out at the gym) and got more involved in my studies. My eating habits deteriorated to a steady diet of high-calorie processed junk food—convenient and cheap was my mantra. Before I knew it, I was carrying around an extra fifty pounds or more. Ironically, I had a part-time job as a personal trainer, which kept me in decent shape despite the extra weight. Happy with my status quo, and promising myself to slim down after the MCAT was over, I started eating whatever and whenever I wanted to—which meant five to seven times a day.

That's when the strangest thing happened. After about a month of this new lifestyle, I noticed that my pants were looser—ten pounds, gone. The muscles remained, but the love handles were disappearing. It wasn't due to stress. What is going on here? I wondered. I was eating more meals per day, and I was exercising a lot less, but my body was looking better. How could this be? I was determined to find out.

At first, I played with my diet to decrease even more body fat. I thought this required eating more carbohydrates (which to me at the time meant processed breads, crackers, and packaged meals) and eating less protein. I was also concentrating less on lifting weights at the gym in favor of aerobic conditioning through running. This new plan created a two-fold problem: the carbs were putting me on a mental and physical roller coaster ride, and the absence of weight training decreased my muscle mass. I was naïve about good protein so I ate steak, cheese, or other easily accessible high-protein foods that were also high in fat. To fix this, I focused on eating even less fat and compensated by loading up on fat-free dishes high in carbohydrates and salt. My weight did not change significantly, but I kept losing muscle mass, and the love handles were reappearing.

4

Then, I refocused my diet to eating leaner proteins like chicken, fish, and nonfat dairy products. This seemed to correct the fat gain and muscle loss, but I was still gulping down a large espresso every day after lunch to avoid the coma-like state I fell into after meals. The carbohydrate rush from the prepared foods I was still eating was making my blood sugar plummet one and a half to two hours after each meal. And to make matters worse, once this stupor passed, I was hungry again and had a hard time concentrating in class. This plan was not working.

My salvation came from my biochemistry classes. They taught me the truth about metabolism, food groups, and my personal machine—how it worked and what fuel it needed to consume for optimal energy. I learned that all carbs are not created equal, and the same was true for fats and proteins. All three food groups have healthy and unhealthy varieties.

I started to concentrate on eating more unprocessed and complex (good) carbohydrates—vegetables, fruit, and whole grains—and avoided simple processed (bad) carbs—mainly sugary foods. Immediately I felt better, but it was not the final formula I was looking for.

I finally tied all of the information together: I added more lean protein, continued eating quality carbs and fat, minimized my salt intake, and ate five to six smaller meals per day. Right away I noticed the difference. I was more alert and felt no fatigue after meals. Quality fuels and more frequent meals were helping to regulate the way my body burned calories. Weeks later I noticed that my muscle tone and mass were returning and were easier to maintain with added weight training and less total exercise.

Finally, I had found the perfect way to eat and exercise while maintaining my health and fitness goals. With this newfound knowledge and proof of its effectiveness, I set out to first learn why these eating habits really worked and then find a way to share my good news.

Knowledge Is Power

This was just the beginning of my dietary sleuthing. Through trial and error, I became convinced that diet, above all, is central to weight management and maintaining health. For me, the exercise maven, it was an eye-opening discovery. But why then do all diets have such miserable track records when it comes to losing weight and keeping it off? I found the answer.

My research has led me to develop an eating program that for the past twenty years has allowed me to maintain my optimum weight and cut my exercise regimen in half while maintaining my ideal fitness level and muscle mass. It may sound trite, but it wasn't until I understood the chemical composition of foods, how they react in my body, and when to eat them that I was able to develop an eating pattern that allowed me to reach my goals. Remember, the secret to losing weight and keeping it off is not just about calorie restriction. It is not as simple as eating low-fat or low-carbohydrate foods. It's about knowledge—knowledge of what to eat, when to eat, and how much to eat.

Be Autonomous

Anyone can eat healthy for a while and lose some weight, but what do the 5–10 percent who do maintain their results have that the rest of us do not? Autonomy: they have created and continue to manage their fitness program on their own. How? They simply know what they are doing and why they are doing it. I am going to help you develop your own personalized Body of Knowledge program that will give you this autonomy.

> THE SECRET TO LOSING WEIGHT AND KEEPING IT OFF IS … KNOWLEDGE OF WHAT TO EAT, WHEN TO EAT, AND HOW MUCH TO EAT.

What you won't find in this book are gimmicks and quick weight-loss schemes. Though I do offer a BOK Accelerated Fat Loss Meal Plan™, trust me, it will not happen overnight. What you will experience, however, is a gradual reduction in your weight and body fat, more muscle tone, robust energy, mental clarity, and a renewed spirit.

When it comes to optimum health, the most important thing you can feed yourself is knowledge. Let's start with a little background in human history and a recap of some of the science you learned in high school. Hang in there; this isn't hard. Think of this as an owner's manual to your most important possession—your healthy body. Knowing how your body responds to foods and activities is fundamental to establishing your autonomy.

The Body: The Ultimate Machine

I'm with Leonardo Da Vinci. The human body is the uncontested ultimate machine on planet earth. Yes, we humans have built incredible, complex machines that are energy efficient and have automated processes. But do they have the ability to manufacture their own fuel, automatically store it, build replacement parts from this fuel, and repair themselves?

This machine worked perfectly for our ancestors. They got up at dawn and went to bed at sunset. They hunted, foraged, traveled, and played to naturally keep in shape. And, most certainly, they ate whatever they came across in small, healthy portions several times a day to ensure survival. These basic instincts never adapted to the fact that we now have an unlimited supply of food, that we actually develop foods that are unhealthy and make them easily accessible, and that we have all sorts of technology and conveniences that minimize our daily activity. We've created a dangerous super-sized, non-nutritional nightmare of a national diet that has led us to our present obesity levels and related medical problems like diabetes and heart disease. We have basically engineered ourselves away from a healthy lifestyle.

Life Changed, Habits Didn't

The truth is we're not that far from the instincts of our ancestors—at least where food is concerned. Too many of us approach the dinner table as if we may not eat again tomorrow, thinking the same way that early man had to, just to survive. And now, America is the fattest nation in the world. Our cups runneth over—and our waistlines are now running over our belts. The most recent statistics show that more than half of all Americans are overweight—10 percent of them by one hundred pounds or more. And these numbers are climbing. Yet other statistics show that, at any given time, half of us are on diets. Obviously, something isn't working.

"Dieting" requires us to ignore the basic needs of our bodies. Food deprivation goes against the grain of natural instincts. By ignoring hunger signals, eliminating foods that our bodies may need, and skipping meals altogether, we are aggravating our instinctual responses to food. This is one of the greatest challenges when it comes to losing weight; most of the time, we are working against our instincts.

Where Did We Come From?

The popular phrase "dust to dust" is still the easiest way to sum up our existence. All living things share the same atoms and molecules from the beginning of life to the end of life: carbon, oxygen, nitrogen, and hydrogen. These elements form the trillions of individual cells that make up the body and the active processes, such as metabolism, that allow us to function. We were designed to absorb nutrients that exist in natural, or unprocessed, foods made up of these same four main elements.

According to recent studies, anthropologists have found that early man ate lean meats, fresh fruit, assorted vegetables, and nuts. Food was naturally available in the environment and naturally provided all of the nutrients that humans needed to run their machines at peak efficiency. Food was not readily available in a refrigerator in the next room—they had to work for it back then. But most importantly, they ate when their body told them to: throughout the day, usually five to seven small meals.

Sometimes food was scarce, and because of that, early man was instinct-driven for survival. Eat it when you find it because you might not be eating tomorrow. The most brilliant natural defense mechanism to ward off starvation was the body's ability to store fat. Fat is high in calories and is an excellent fuel. It is also compact and can store more calories in smaller spaces throughout the body than carbohydrates and proteins.

In the early years of human development, fat was the wonder fuel. Fat supplied energy for the constant physical activity required in the days of hunting and gathering. There was little opportunity for fat to collect around midsections or

> EARLY MAN ATE LEAN MEATS, FRESH FRUIT, ASSORTED VEGETABLES, AND NUTS.

anywhere else on the body in large quantities. As time moved on and agriculture developed, societies depended less and less on hunting and gathering. Starvation became a concern only in the years when harvests were bad. As we became more "civilized" and our crops provided more food than we needed to survive, things began to change. What was genetically programmed into us to ensure our existence was beginning to threaten our health and very survival.

The other factor that now contributes to our collective weight and health problems is inactivity. Early man had to work hard to gather the fruits, vegetables, nuts, and lean wild game that made up his diet. Primitive man ate very few "empty" calories—there were no cupcakes, potato chips, or candy bars to be gathered in the forest!

ALL THINGS BIG AND SMALL

Simply put, macronutrients (macro = big nutrients) have a dual role: they are building blocks for our bodies and also act as fuel to keep it running. Micronutrients (micro = small nutrients) are exactly what their name states, smaller parts of our machine necessary to run important processes like our metabolism.

Macronutrients	Micronutrients
Carbohydrates	Vitamins
Protein	Minerals
Fats	

However, today we live in a time of limitless food choices and availability. We drive cars, take elevators, sit at desks, and view exercise as work. Our goal now is to untwist what has gone wrong in our lifestyles and get back to the way things should be.

The Big Picture: It's All about Energy

The human body is like a chemical factory. Thousands of chemicals are churning and mixing and reacting inside of us. And the power source for this factory is energy. The energy needed to power the body comes in the form of calories—a word every dieter is very familiar with. Our calories are either burned or stored for use as energy on an as-needed basis. But energy doesn't like to sit around waiting to be called into action. Unlike energy that waits to be turned on in your home and flows only in one direction, the energy that powers your body is in a constant state of flux—it flows both ways depending on your need to either burn it or store it.

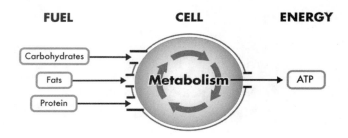

Most people assume that the three types of fuel that make up our food—carbohydrates, fat, and protein—directly supply the body with the energy it needs to function. Not so. All types of energy need a vehicle, a way to move around. Unlike the electrical wiring in your home, the energy in your body uses molecules to move around. An important molecule known as adenosine triphosphate (ATP) is the battery that keeps your machine going. Think of the three fuels you eat as three grades of gasoline that produce different amounts of energy and think of ATP as a battery on wheels that takes that energy (a.k.a. calories) produced by the three fuels to wherever it is needed. The three fuels all produce different amounts of ATP, but fat produces much more than carbohydrates or protein. Translated, this fundamental biochemical fact means fat produces more calories (or ATP) per gram than its cousins, protein and carbohydrates (carbs):

1 gram of **protein**	= **4 calories**
1 gram of **carbohydrate**	= **4 calories**
1 gram of **fat**	= **9 calories**

Energy Basics

In a perfect biochemical world, our bodies would take in the precise amount of calories we need to burn to keep our bodies at their ideal weights. For too many of us, this doesn't happen. Most of us eat more calories than our bodies require, and excess calories go straight to the storage bin (which is usually around your waistline or hips).

> ENERGY = CALORIES
> *ATP* IS THE CALORIE *CARRIER*

> WANT TO SEE WHAT HAPPENS WHEN YOU EAT AND RUN?
> WE DID THE MATH FOR YOU ON THE WEB SITE.

The simple equation of burn more energy than you consume is central to any reputable weight-loss program. It doesn't matter if you eat pounds of food or no food, eat every fifteen minutes or once a day, eat only grapefruit and egg whites, meat and potatoes, or coffee and doughnuts. In order to lose weight you must burn more energy than you consume. However—and this is at the heart of a smart weight-management program—there are ways to consume calories that will enable you to burn energy more quickly. And, there are foods and food combinations that are used more efficiently by the body and are less likely to turn into fat. Later I am going to show you how to combine this knowledge with efficient exercise so that you won't have to worry about counting every calorie at every meal or focus on the scale ever again.

Food as Building Blocks

Now you know that the way to burn calories most efficiently has a lot to do with the quality, quantities, and combinations of the three fuels—carbohydrates, protein, and fat—that we consume. Our bodies use each fuel in the foods we eat in a different way, so varying the percentage of one fuel or combining two fuels will produce different results. The three fuels also play different roles in building and maintaining the bones, muscles, and organs in our body. Yes, you really are what you eat. The compositions of the fuels that give us energy to live and function are also the building blocks of our bodies. And because both the human body and food supplied by Mother Nature are composed of the same organic compounds—carbohydrates, protein, and fat—then it only makes sense that we maintain our bodily structures with the intended building blocks designed by Mother Nature.

Carbohydrates

Carbohydrates play a major role in energy creation and regulation, but they are limited in their structural contribution. They don't directly build the mortar and bricks of our bodies' construction, but they do affect the quality of the construction. For example, they protect our stomach linings from the harsh acid environment and help lubricate our joints. They also make up one of the three basic parts of DNA, which is what our genes are made of.

Carbohydrates also play an important role in the regulation and release of the hormones serotonin and insulin. Serotonin levels can affect your mood and mental clarity. Insulin is one of the key players in the fat storage game. All of these starring roles—energy production, quality of construction, and regulation—make carbohydrates like a quarterback on a football team. They are key players, and they also make some important decisions in the game.

Protein

When it comes to safeguarding our structure, protein plays the biggest role of all. If carbs are like a quarterback, protein is like the rest of the team, plus the coaches,

> YES, YOU REALLY ARE WHAT YOU EAT.

recruiters, fans—even the stadium. Protein's structural contribution to the body is well known (e.g., muscles and bones), but what is more essential is its job as the main chemical component of *enzymes*. Enzymes are vital to the body because they run all of our life-sustaining chemical reactions.

ENZYMES—YOUR BODY'S ASSEMBLY LINES

At this moment, every vital biochemical reaction occurring inside of us is dependent upon the 10,000 different enzymes swimming around in our bodies.

Enzymes are not only made of protein, they are also the only substance capable of breaking down the protein that we eat and then using it to build all the protein structures in our body. This "rate of reaction" is essential for life because any enzyme deficiencies or dysfunctions can result in serious or even life-threatening health problems. Like assembly line workers, enzymes can also add new elements to existing parts or break down structures for other purposes, like growth and healing from injuries. Problems with or a lack of certain enzymes can cause problems or even serious illnesses; learn more about this on the web site.

Protein is the major component in such bodily structures as muscles, tendons, bones, hair, and internal organs. It is also the main chemical component of hormones, blood cells, antibodies, and important chemical messengers (like insulin). Growth, reproduction, metabolic processes, and even emotional responses are dependent on protein.

Fat

When it comes to maintaining our physical structure, fat is vital to basic survival. As much as we try to rid our diets of fat, without it the most basic structure in our bodies—the cell—could not exist. Fat's main job is to keep cells and us alive. Fat molecules make up cell walls, which are responsible for keeping cells intact. Our life processes all occur in watery environments, which need the natural repelling properties of fats and oils to keep everything in its proper place. Simply put, the oily cell walls keep the good watery things in and the bad ones out. You may never look at the olive oil in your Italian salad dressing the same way again!

The male and female sex hormones (testosterone and estrogen) are also predominantly constructed of a fat derivative. And fats form the basis of myelin, a substance that coats nerve cells, like the plastic insulation around an electrical wire. Cerebral palsy and multiple sclerosis are conditions caused by damage to the fatty myelin covering around nerves.

> FAT'S MAIN JOB IS TO KEEP CELLS AND US ALIVE.

Unfortunately, fat gets a bad rap for being the lazy building block. It snuggles up under the skin, forming that infamous spare tire that develops around the waist. But unlike protein, fat prefers to burn itself off as fuel. Though fat's role as a structural requirement is relatively simple, its role in the makeup of the food we eat is quite complex. The average consumer is well aware of the endless arguments over the benefits and evils of saturated, unsaturated, polyunsaturated, monounsaturated, and trans-fats. Unfortunately much of the truth about fat has been misinterpreted or misunderstood.

CHOLESTEROL: FAT'S BUILDING BUDDY

Cholesterol is many things (both good and bad), but the fat you eat and the cholesterol in your body are two different things. Cholesterol is a type of modified fat, but it is not a type of fat used for fuel—cholesterol has no calories. Like dietary fat, however, it has an important role. Along with dietary fat it helps form a protective coating around cell walls. It also helps build hormones, like testosterone, progesterone, and estrogen. The problem with cholesterol is that we can get too much of it. Because it is essential, the body has the ability to make the amount of cholesterol it needs on its own from fat supplies. Too much cholesterol is bad enough, but too much fat and cholesterol can collect in our blood vessels, and this is a proven lethal combination that contributes to our high rate of heart disease.

Shellfish, such as crab, lobster, and shrimp, are great lean protein sources, but they contain some of the highest concentrations of cholesterol in their cell walls. The meat in shellfish is low in calories only because of cholesterol's inability to be recognized by the body as a fuel. Even though shellfish is a great source of low-fat protein, you may want to check your cholesterol level if you eat it more than two to three times a week.

Adding Up the Three Fuels

I hope that you are starting to see why any diet that minimizes or cuts out an entire food or fuel group just doesn't make sense. Once you learn how to effectively combine the three fuels and learn how to manage your intake, you will no longer make your food choices solely on taste or convenience or impulse. If you look at food as fuel and building blocks and select unprocessed varieties that provide all the benefits a healthy, fit body requires, then your weight and fitness goals will be within reach.

> ANY DIET THAT MINIMIZES OR CUTS OUT AN ENTIRE FOOD OR FUEL GROUP JUST DOESN'T MAKE SENSE.

I want to stress that if you eat for your body's needs, you don't have to sacrifice anything in the way of taste, texture, or eye appeal. I'll show you how to make creative choices to a point where eating what you want and eating what you need will become one and the same. Now that we've covered the basics of how food creates energy and provides the building blocks for all of your body parts, it's time to move on to your body's need for another kind of energy, the kind you exert—exercise.

Exercise: Make Your Workouts Work for You

Exercise is as essential to a healthy body as eating the right food. It is a critical part of the process that maintains our fitness levels and basic bodily structures. First and foremost, exercise helps keep our hearts strong and our arteries flowing. Exercise also stimulates the calcium-building process in our bones, so we can slow the bone-thinning, debilitating disease of old age: osteoporosis.

When done properly, exercise helps keep the slippery fluid in our joints flowing and helps maintain healthy cartilage, thus easing the joint friction that leads to arthritis. So exercise benefits the heart, arteries, bones, and joints, but that's not all. Most importantly, exercise helps keep our muscles conditioned by building and maintaining their mass. Maintaining healthy muscle mass means continued strength and the ability to maintain your ideal weight. The more muscle mass you acquire and maintain, the more calories you burn throughout the day. This is because more muscle equals better metabolism, which uses more fuel, even when you are at rest.

> MORE MUSCLE = BETTER METABOLISM.

Exercise keeps muscles toned and helps fight the effects of aging—a sagging backside, flabby upper arms, and the dimpling-effect of cellulite. Exercise is essential to our staying power. It helps us take the stairs easier, walk or run farther, breathe more efficiently, and increases our energy. There is even scientific evidence to prove that exercise is a mood elevator, depression fighter, and an overall age extender. But, you must be asking by now, what about weight loss? Exercise is synonymous with weight loss, right? Well, get ready for another surprise.

Exercise is the Other Energy

For most people who decide that they want (or need) to lose weight, the knee-jerk response is "I've got to get to the gym." Few of these people look forward to scheduled exercise and view it as a painful step to weight loss. Many people mistakenly believe that exercise is more important than a healthy diet when it comes to any type of weight management.

> EXERCISE IS MOST IMPORTANT IN *MAINTAINING* YOUR WEIGHT AND HEALTH.

It is our eating habits that profoundly affect our personal well-being and longevity and act as the primary force for shedding body fat and regulating metabolism. Exercise burns calories, but it is most important in *maintaining* your weight. In the absence of a properly managed diet, exercise alone will at best just slow fat production and storage. So if you want lasting results and better overall health proper exercise is essential.

EXERCISE IS ENERGY EXERTED

I like to think of exercise as the other energy—the energy we exert in order to burn more calories. Like the energy we take in (food), the energy we put out (exercise) is a matter of quantity and quality. Remember how ATP is produced from the three fuel groups—fats, carbohydrates, and protein—to supply energy to its needed destination? Exercise uses up a lot of ATP, so when more is needed, fat cells are called on to produce a new supply, thus indirectly reducing fat stores.

Quality, Not Quantity

The biggest problem with exercise is that most people look at it like a chore, something they have to do. It doesn't have to be this way. You can exercise effectively in less time and with less effort than you think. Different exercises produce different results.

Whether your goals require fat loss, muscle toning, muscle building, aerobic conditioning, cross-training, or a combination of them all, your physical efforts should be specific to your goals and need not be excessive. Too many people learn too late that more exercise is not better. They exercise more than they should, or perform maneuvers that are not effective in helping them reach their goals. This limits their achievements, creates disappointment, can cause injuries, and ultimately contributes to the high dropout rate.

The key to an effective exercise and weight-loss program involves three parameters: repetitions, technique, and breathing. Huffing and puffing programs and "no pain, no gain" thinking are a thing of the past. Research has shown that results in any area of exercise can be achieved with a lot less time and effort than traditional physical training programs.

The Dynamic Duo: The Combined Power of Diet and Exercise

Fact: you can essentially produce any change in your body by using a combination of diet modifications and different physical training techniques. Reducing your caloric intake while burning more calories will obviously help increase your weight loss odds, but there's more to it than that. Here are some encouraging examples:

1. Did you know that your metabolism is designed to be fueled every two to three hours? Yes, you can manage your weight easier and have better overall health by eating smaller meals five to seven times a day.

2. Medical research shows that the most effective tool for living longer and enjoying better health is eating less. Animals that were allowed to overeat at every meal had more heart disease, diabetes, cancer than the ones that simply ate less. And the one who ate less lived 20 percent longer!

3. Did you know that your metabolism burns at a faster rate for many hours after most conditioning exercises are finished? That means a larger portion of your next meal will be burned off instead of being stored in your body as extra calories if you exercise before.

4. Timing between exercises is important as well as eating particular foods before or after exercise because both can make it easier to create and maintain muscle mass. This means less total exercise is required, creating a less stressful fitness cycle

that constantly feeds off itself to ensure that you reach your goals and maintain them once they are achieved.

Not only will you be able to create your own diet and exercise program after reading Parts 2 and 3, but in Part 4, Putting it All Together, you will have the option to choose from five different real-life examples that have sample eating and exercise programs provided for each one. I encourage you to enjoy yourself in the process. You are about to take charge of your health and fitness in a way you never have before, with more quality information than you have ever had from one source.

Free Your Mind and Your Body Will Follow

Apatient of mine named Jim came to me as a typical middle-aged man juggling too many balls in the air between his family and work. He first complained about his inability to exercise since he had less energy, less time, and painful joints. He would wake up at five in the morning and hit the weights before work, skip breakfast, and then have lunch during meetings, eating whatever they served (usually takeout). By three he was pounding down several cups of coffee to stave off fatigue and taking ibuprofen for his knees, which ached after sitting all day in one position. When he came home, he had to have a few beers or cocktails to "wind down." By the time dinner was ready he was famished and wolfed down the usual he-man helping of food that he had been praised for eating as a young man. Then he was off to watch television with the family, but this wasn't quality time since he would pass out an hour after eating. Hours later, after his wife would wake him and tell him it was time to go to bed, he would have a hard time getting to sleep and then feel exhausted when the alarm went off at five again the next morning.

Jim was also a borderline diabetic and taking oral medication to control his blood sugar. He came to me desperate for help, and we put together his personalized BOK program. He was able to untwist his unhealthy lifestyle and correct the problems he had been developing since childhood. First he started to feel more energy eating five meals per day instead of two. He made many excuses in the beginning about eating this frequently, but found there were always possibilities to catch a quick snack (even if he had to excuse himself from a meeting to "go to the men's room" and eat a piece of fruit, small yogurt, or protein bar). He also noticed that the amount of alcohol he was drinking to wind down was not only wreaking havoc with his blood sugar but the disinhibition or "buzz" that it provided really triggered a type of mindless speed eating that made him gorge at dinner.

After changing his eating habits, he noticed that a snack at 3:30 or 4:00 completely erased the feeling of hunger and anxiety that drove him to reach for his cocktails in the first place—to a point where he lost any need to wind down at all and changed his drinking habits to an occasional glass or two of red wine. In fact, he found himself interacting with his wife and children more, taking the time to discuss their day and school activities. Dinner became a tranquil event and not a race. Now his family walks after dinner, providing the opportunity for even more time together while they continue to add to their new health and fitness goals. And, during these walks he found a group of gentlemen who would work out during lunch or after work downtown near his office. The steady weight loss not only allowed him to eventually get off of the medication for his diabetes, but also alleviated the load on his knees, to the point that he could even catch a few pick-up basketball games with the neighborhood kids.

Others do not always get to enjoy a simple, straight-forward program and sustainable results like Jim did though. I had another special patient named Tracy, whom you'll get to know later in this book. She followed her own BOK program too and physically lost a lot of weight, but then wasn't able to handle the weight loss emotionally. She gained back almost a hundred pounds. Once she told me the shocking truth behind her emotional weight gain, I was able to help her. It took some effort, but Tracy was able to understand and face the reasons why she regained the weight, and she eventually won her battle.

It appears that for each of us, there are no absolutes in the world of diet and exercise. True weight management is a lifestyle unique to each person, but the interaction between our mind and body seems to be consistent for everyone—like Tracy discovered. The body and the mind do not function separately or independent of one another.

Rather, they are wholly interdependent. The mind has amazing powers over the body, and much of that influence is good. Your mind can push your body in the direction of good health and successful weight management or push it in the opposite direction. On the other hand, your body's overall health can support mental clarity and better decisions or influence bad habits that lead to unhealthy choices. Consider those days when you are so mentally or emotionally drained that you are incapable of any physical activity at all. Conversely, think of the difficulty you have in maintaining mental focus and productivity after a full day of physical activity—or after eating a bacon cheeseburger and fries.

Identifying the Obstacles

Popular media along with many scientific studies have pointed to our physical failings as the cause of the rising obesity rate in the United States. We don't eat right and we don't exercise enough. Is this a physical failing—or is it a mental one?

> FORGET THE WORD "WILLPOWER."

Think back again to those common everyday obstacles we run into during our quest for health and fitness. In reality, this is what is behind the majority of setbacks and the high attrition rate in weight management. The temptation of ever-present junk food makes you cave too often. You may skip exercise because of a few stiff muscles, or in your frustration to break a weight loss plateau, you just want to give up. There are too many obstacles, and they all affect us differently.

Some people have dysfunctional eating habits or what is clinically known as an eating disorder. These problems range in severity from overeating excessively and gaining five to ten pounds over the holidays, to bingeing on weekends, to more severe problems such as bulimia and anorexia. What is more alarming is that these problems are more common than you might think. I will go so far as to say that anyone who continually struggles with their weight is suffering from some type of eating dysfunction, addiction, or disorder.

Overcoming the Obstacles: The Positive Picture

Physical obstacles like soreness, burning, stiffness, cramping, and pla-teaus do get in the way of everyone's fitness goals, and I will show you simple ways to navigate through them or avoid them altogether. Oth-er obstacles are not as obvious though. Recent medical studies prove that certain mental and social issues contribute to a large percentage of poor diet and fitness outcomes. Without addressing those issues you can never win the sadistic game of lose-gain-lose-gain. There is also new scientific evidence that shows how basic brain functions sup-port some of these bad habits and how the mind tries to override your intellectual ability to defeat them.

Fear not—there are ways to get over all these hurdles so you can attain your goals. I'll help you identify your particular obstacles, con-nect with their origins in Part 5, and once and for all correct them at their sources. Understanding the obstacles and your mind's reaction to them will give you the knowledge and power to overcome them. Forget the word "willpower." It isn't in my health and fitness vocabu-lary, and it shouldn't be in yours. Once the hidden reasons behind a particular setback are discovered, they lose their detrimental effect on your efforts. Your machine will no longer be controlling you; you will be back online and in charge.

Welcome to BOKsystems. You will use these new tools for your self-discovery. And, combined with my eating and exercise plans, you will be able to form your own Body of Knowledge program.

Let's get started.

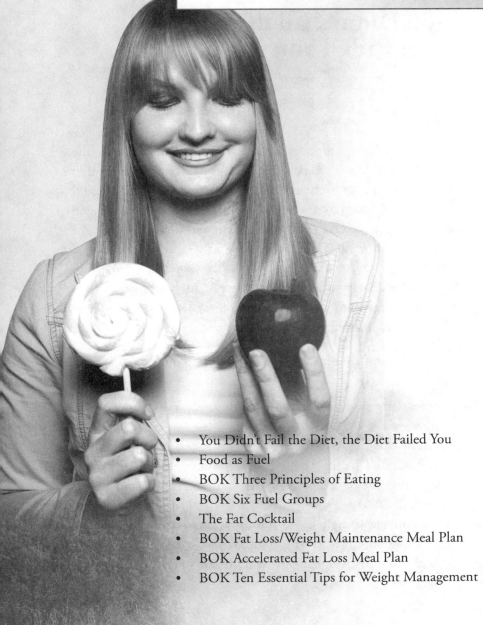

PART 2

FOOD AND EATING HABITS

- You Didn't Fail the Diet, the Diet Failed You
- Food as Fuel
- BOK Three Principles of Eating
- BOK Six Fuel Groups
- The Fat Cocktail
- BOK Fat Loss/Weight Maintenance Meal Plan
- BOK Accelerated Fat Loss Meal Plan
- BOK Ten Essential Tips for Weight Management

27

You Didn't Fail the Diet, the Diet Failed You

Every new program, product, or expert claims that they have the right answer. Many are popular, gimmick-driven programs that require strict adherence to their rules and supplements or fad diets renowned for their followers and testimonials. Almost all end up being infamous for their success in the short term and disappointment in the long term. The truth is that only you know your true goals, wants, and needs. You need to find your own answers and take ownership of the best choices for you. My goal is to provide you with enough information so you can answer these questions and make your own decisions—decisions that make sense for your lifestyle and produce the results you want.

The How and Why

I believe that any sustainable, healthy eating plan must follow three basic rules:

1. A healthy eating plan must work in the real world: eating in, out, or on the run; eating alone, with friends, or at parties; eating freshly prepared meals or commercially prepared foods.
2. A sustainable eating plan must offer a variety of choices. Nobody is going to stick with a gimmick—fat free, all protein, no carbs, costly supplements, and prepared meals—for very long.

3. Your eating plan must make sense to you. You need to understand the "what, how, and why"—what foods will give you the results you want, how much and how often to eat them, and why your plan will produce those results so you can maintain a healthy weight on your own.

> GIMMICK-DRIVEN PROGRAMS...OR FAD DIETS...END UP BEING INFAMOUS FOR THEIR SUCCESS IN THE SHORT-TERM AND DISAPPOINTMENT IN THE LONG-TERM.

I used these rules to develop the BOK Three Principles of Eating™, the foundation of my eating management and weight-management program. These principles of successful eating are simple, straightforward, and based on scientific findings. The key is to properly match the best quantity and quality of protein, carbohydrate, and fat, then eat them at the best times throughout the day.

BOK Three Principles of Eating:
Principle 1: How much to eat
Principle 2: How often to eat
Principle 3: What to eat

These principles are designed to help you reach your goals and keep them by eating in an enjoyable, satisfying, and healthy way. And you'll never feel that you are sacrificing food because you will never feel hungry. Why? Because you'll be eating more often. Furthermore, the BOK Three Principles of Eating will train your taste buds and stomach to recognize the best foods, the best portion size for each food, and the best fuel to consume at specific times throughout the day.

In this section of the book I will also teach you about the BOK Six Fuel Groups™, a food classification system that allows you to mix and match healthy food choices. While learning what to eat, you will also learn about the different qualities of foods and how to minimize your time in the kitchen and at the grocery store. Finally, I will offer two specific eating programs that are designed to simplify your eating habits: the first is for fat loss and weight maintenance, and the second is an accelerated fat loss program to help you meet your goals at a faster but sensible pace.

Most dieters spend their lifetimes in a battle with food, chasing fad diets without really understanding the relationship between food and weight management. I'll help you put a stop to this madness.

Remember what you learned earlier in this book: food provides building blocks for your body, but it fuels the body too. Think of your body as a top performance race car that requires quality parts and needs a specific blend of fuels to run fast and efficiently for a long time. In the end, permanent weight loss is all about endurance—endurance in the human race for longevity and good health. But, before we explore the BOK Three Principles of Eating and the BOK Six Fuel Groups, it is very important that you have a good, basic understanding of how food fuels the body. With your newfound knowledge about food, you will be able to make smarter decisions and stick with a lifelong healthy eating program.

Food as Fuel

All the systems in your body work together like any company to maximize production and efficiency. Think of your brain as performing the role of Chief Executive Officer (CEO), managing all the operations within your body, making the smart decisions to keep your machine running as efficiently as possible and feeding it the right fuels in the right amounts at the right times. Like any good CEO, your brain needs to use its resources effectively. As was explained in Part 1, your body requires specific building blocks to help maintain its structure and functions. When you use a smart eating strategy, the same building blocks work together to help you fuel your machine effectively. Let's take a look at the resources you have at your disposal to best fuel and run your body's business.

Carbohydrates: The Workforce

Never underestimate the power of carbs. This fuel not only does most of the work, but also influences the overall operations of all three fuels. A simple carbohydrate has a far greater influence on your weight-management goals than any other fuel source. Carbohydrates possess most of the power dictating whether you will burn fuel or store it. Carbohydrate-containing foods even influence the way you think. Of all the fuels, carbohydrates need careful management, but the effort is well worth it.

If you ingest too many carbs at once, they will cause a flood of the hormone *insulin*, which locks down fat and sends it to the fat cells for storage. It's important to note that fat conversion is a lopsided chemical reaction. Once insulin is released, it will store that extra fat we do not burn and then convert extra carbs and protein that is not utilized into more fat too. But when we are exercising to burn off the excess fat and our carbohydrate stores dwindle, we cannot reverse this chemical re-

> A SIMPLE CARBOHYDRATE HAS A FAR GREATER INFLUENCE ON YOUR WEIGHT-MANAGEMENT GOALS THAN ANY OTHER FUEL SOURCE.

action to replenish the carbohydrates. Insulin acts as the supervisor, ensuring that our bodies do not convert fats back into carbohydrates to burn as fuel! Like me, I hope that once you know the secret of this unfair one-way chemical reaction, you will put carbohydrate management high on your priority list. You can skip ahead to the section "Insulin: The Storage Hormone" to learn more about insulin's effects on fat storage.

UNFAIR BIOCHEMISTRY

Fat Conversion

CARBOHYDRATES→→→→→**YES**→→→→→ FAT
CARBOHYDRATES←←←←←**NO**←←←←← FAT

Fact: The more carbs you eat, the more storage hormone you body releases.

But, because all carbs are not created equal, you must also pay attention to the quality of carbs that you choose, too. The type of carbs you eat will also affect insulin release. Scientifically speaking, there are only two general types of carbohydrates: *simple carbohydrates* and *complex carbohydrates.*

Complex carbohydrates have one broad category: polysaccharides, or many (poly) individual sugar (saccharide) molecules hooked together. They come in all different lengths and combinations. Overall, complex carbs should always be your first carb choice at mealtime because they enter your bloodstream slower and thus release less insulin. This makes complex carbs a better quality fuel for weight management and better health. But do not fixate on them. Simple carbs are necessary too for things like exercise performance and mental functions.

Simple carbohydrates have two categories: disaccharides (two sugar molecules) and monosaccharides (one sugar molecule). The monosaccharides go by the names glucose, fructose, and galactose. The disaccharides—maltose (found in beer), sucrose (table sugar), and lactose (found in milk)—are just different combinations of the three monosaccharide sugars.

Now that you have passed Saccharide 101, let's apply your new knowledge to everyday foods that we all recognize. Before the birth of the carbohydrate-bashing high-protein diets, carbs were commonly known by their three friendly subsets: sugars, starches, and fiber. All of these foods have complex and/or simple carbohydrates in them, although the amounts vary. So it is both the food type and the makeup that matter when it comes to your diet.

The Familiar Faces of Carbs

1. **Sugars**, or simple carbohydrates, are found in honey, milk products, certain vegetables, fruit, and other processed carbohydrate products, such as high fructose syrups and ordinary table sugar.

2. **Starches**, or complex carbohydrates, are in legumes (e.g., kidney beans), grains, vegetables, and fruit.

3. **Fiber**, another complex carbohydrate, is found in whole grains, legumes, vegetables, and fruits.

Sugar Highs and Lows

Refined sugar is not a creation of Mother Nature. She does, however, provide sugar in unprocessed foods, such as fruits, honey, milk products, and certain vegetables. The difference in how your body processes refined sugar compared to sugars that exist in natural foods is revealed in the popularized glycemic index (GI). Since not all simple or complex carbs are processed the same way in our bodies, the GI provides a scale that shows how each food item containing carbohydrates compares to pure glucose absorption—a GI value of 100.

The lower the GI, the less sugar is absorbed into your bloodstream (and usually less insulin released) after eating a particular food item. Table sugar, white flour, and almost all the other processed carbs have a higher glycemic index (70 and above), while some fruits and most vegetables have a lower glycemic index. For example, apples that contain "fruit sugars" and other varieties only have a GI range of 30–40. The complex carbohydrates in fruits and vegetables are responsible for this difference.

> THE GI PROVIDES A SCALE THAT SHOWS HOW EACH FOOD ITEM CONTAINING CARBOHYDRATES COMPARES TO PURE GLUCOSE.

The problem with the GI is that it is most useful for scientific research. The Glycemic *Load* (GL) is a better way to select carbohydrates if you are watching your weight (and for less insulin released). The GL is the GI multiplied by the amount of carbohydrate per serving. For example, carrots have a high GI, but lower GL because they contain a lot of water and fiber. You can search for the GI and GL of your favorite foods on the web site.

GLYCEMIC INDEX AND GLYCEMIC LOAD RANGES

Glycemic Index Range	Glycemic Load Range
Low GI = 55 or less	Low GL = 10 or less
Medium GI = 56–69	Medium GL = 11–19
High GI = 70 or more	High GL = 20 or more

Recommended Glycemic Load per Day

Low GL < 80

High GL > 120

Fructose is unique because it is not really detected by the glycemic index since the test is sensitive only to glucose—the common sugar in all carbohydrates, simple and complex. Fructose's inherent low glycemic index has made it a very popular sweetener in snacks, prepared foods, and protein bars, but new research shows that it's a pay-now or pay-later situation. When fructose enters the bloodstream, it is sent to the liver, where it is converted into glucose. Eventually a similar glycemic load and total sugar metabolism is delivered to your body.

Light on the Starch

This broad category is mainly made up of vegetables, grains, and legumes, but many fruits also contain the starchy polysaccharides. They are all complex carbohydrates, although some can have a rather high glycemic index. As always, it depends on the amount of fiber they contain and the processing that takes place. While eating processed wheat products is not as good as eating tomatoes, choosing the whole grain types is a better choice overall. For example, eat whole grain pasta (which contains more fiber) instead of pasta made with enriched flour.

Potatoes and other "tubers" get a bad rap because their glycemic index is quite high. These root vegetables are the carbohydrate storage bins of the plant world. It's not the concentration of carbs that is the problem; it's how we prepare them. In general, raw is better than cooked for any and all unprocessed carbohydrate-containing foods. The heat generated during cooking breaks down the strong chemical bonds that hook complex carbohydrates together and make them work so well for weight management. Carbohydrates from cooked vegetables have a higher GI and enter the bloodstream faster than uncooked veggies because the long complex carb chains break down into more simple sugars during the cooking process.

Of course, eating a raw potato or yam is not enticing, and raw rice, wheat, or corn is really not an option. However, carrots, broccoli, celery, and other fiber-filled vegetables are great raw and crunchy. Eaten raw, you can be sure that the carbs are at their lowest possible GI, entering your system in a slow-release mode and keeping insulin at its lowest possible level (not to mention better vitamin and mineral absorption).

Be Fiber Optic

Fiber is about as close as we can get to a dream food that contains little to no calories. Fiber is a complex carbohydrate that remains essentially unaltered in its journey through the body, which should make it another carbohydrate of choice. Your best fiber choices are vegetables, fruits, legumes, and whole grains.

Fiber falls into two scientific categories: insoluble and soluble.

Insoluble fiber does not attract or dissolve in liquid of any type. Bran is a great example of insoluble fiber. This type of fiber can pass through your body without being digested—virtually unchanged and unaltered. It keeps your gastrointestinal system clean, healthy, and moving.

Soluble fiber has a different advantage. It can absorb liquids, which means that your stomach will register more bulk from fewer calories, especially when it soaks up some of the contents in your stomach. Furthermore, certain soluble fiber has been shown to attract and trap fats. Like cleaning up an offshore oil spill, fiber from unprocessed foods or over-the-counter supplements, such as psyllium, can reduce the overall fat absorption into your bloodstream. If you drink these supplements for regularity, do so after your biggest meal and take advantage of this extra benefit.

In the end, the smart choice is easy. Stick to unprocessed complex carbs with fiber to keep your machine running better and longer.

Protein: The Warehouse, Machinery, and Equipment

Protein is rarely burned as fuel, but carbs and fat cannot do their jobs without it. Protein is our main building block and keeps the fires stoked and metabolism moving. Its smaller components, amino acids, not only act as the bricks and mortar for your entire machine, they are part of the fuel-burning cycle itself. Certain amino acids are involved in vital chemical reactions, where they assist carbs and fat in the production of ATP (see the Metabolism – Exercise Connection in part 3). Without them, we could not burn fat. Amino acids are classified as either essential or nonessential. We obtain essential amino acids from the food we eat, and our bodies produce the nonessential amino acids.

> AMINO ACIDS ... ARE PART OF THE FUEL-BURNING CYCLE.

NATURALLY OCCURRING AMINO ACIDS

The body can make only thirteen of the amino acids, which are known as the nonessential amino acids. They are called nonessential because the body does not need to extract them from the food we eat. There are nine essential amino acids that are obtained only from food and not made in the body.

From Our Bodies (nonessential)
Asparagine
Aspartic
Cysteine
Cystine
Glutamic
Glutamine
Glycine
Histidine*
Hydroxylysine
Hydroxyproline
Proline
Serine
Tyrosine

From Our Foods (essential)
Arginine
AcidIsoleucine
Leucine
Lysine
Acid Methionine
Phenylalanine
Threonine
Tryptophan
Valine

*Histidine is considered "semi-essential"

Animal Versus Vegetable

In the final analysis, protein selection comes down to a matter of preference: animal or vegetable. Of course, the main problem with eating protein, at least animal protein, is the amount and type of fat that accompanies it. But that does not necessarily make animal protein a taboo because there are plenty of low-fat choices out there to keep us amply satisfied and well nourished. Any mammal, bird, fish, or even reptile will do, since most of these creatures have a similar protein makeup to humans (thus a better amino acid match). I still can't believe how easy it is to go to the grocery store and buy a bag of frozen boneless-skinless chicken breasts, tuna steaks, peeled shrimp, prepackaged "extra lean" meats, egg whites in cartons, as well as a plethora of low-fat and nonfat dairy products.

The key to great protein quality is to choose an animal variety that has been fed as natural a diet as possible. If it is free-range chicken, grass-fed beef, or fresh-caught salmon, the type of fat differs as well as the amount in the meat. The blood chemistries of grass-fed cows have been tested, and not only do they have a lower amount of saturated fat than the corn-fed variety, but they also have a higher amount of healthy omega-3 polyunsaturated fats (found mainly in fish).

Vegetarians and Complementary Protein

Because there is no one vegetable source that contains all of the essential amino acids we need in our daily diet, vegetarians need to consume protein from a variety of sources to ensure adequate amino acid intake. At one time it was believed that in order to consume complete protein in a vegetarian diet, complementary proteins needed to be eaten together in each meal. Beans and rice, peanut butter and whole grain bread, or soy and vegetables were considered some of the combinations that would facilitate the absorption of the necessary essential amino acids. The rule of thumb has since changed, and vegetarians can focus on consuming all of the necessary amino acids throughout the course of a day by varying their meal choices and even using protein supplements.

If you depend solely on plants for protein, you will have to eat a variety of different foods in order to ensure you are getting your daily allotment of essential amino acids. Also, calorie-for-calorie, plants contain less protein than animals, so plan your meals carefully to ensure you are getting enough protein each day.

Don't get me wrong. I am not knocking the vegetarian lifestyle. In fact, I admire it. I just love a nice steak once in a while. Vegetarianism is quite healthy due to the simple fact that it provides more fiber, natural vitamins, and minerals. Aside from the limited protein sources and more challenging meal planning, vegetarians tend to eat less, live longer, and enjoy better health than the average carnivore—something you cannot ignore and I most definitely support.

Fat: Essential Overhead

Fat is most definitely the most efficient of the three fuels. One tablespoon of butter delivers 102 calories and one tablespoon of olive oil delivers 120 calories.

There are two urban myths regarding fat:

1. Fat helps fill you up.

2. Fat makes food taste better.

To put these ideas in true perspective, answer this question: will downing a few tablespoons of pure butter or oil actually fill you up? Of course not. Fats, in their pure chemical form, will not make food taste better either. Our taste buds only register sweet, salt, sour, and bitter taste sensations. Check out the facts about your tongue in the "Fat Cocktail" section.

Taste and smell are interconnected senses, and *aromas* in foods are picked up by both of them. So what does fat contribute? Although many healthy fats (plant oils) contain natural aromas and less healthy fats (butter) contain artificial flavoring or additives such as salt that you can taste, the fat chemical itself contributes only to the consistency of foods and how ingredients blend together. It does not directly stimulate any of your taste buds. Pure fats and oils produce a sensation referred to as "mouth feel"—the richer, smoother, moister feeling that it adds to certain dishes. Herbs, spices, and oils that contain aromas (like virgin olive oil) are really the only things that can give your meals more taste. So unless that slippery feeling in your mouth is a high priority, reach for the spice rack to add more taste instead of adding an entire stick of butter.

My advice is to select and use the fats you like cautiously. A little butter or cream cheese on your toast is actually not a bad thing. The small addition of fat or the natural amount in some foods will help slow the absorption of carbohydrates into the bloodstream, thus decreasing the insulin response. For health purposes, however, you should always go for the unsaturated fats—for example, monounsaturates, found in olive oil and almonds, and polyunsaturates, found in safflower oil and walnuts.

As for fast and hard rules about fat choice and daily amounts, they do not have to be as strict as you may think. Just remember that at the end of the day your heart, arteries, or waistline will know (and eventually show) the difference.

FAT FACTS

For the benefit of a healthy heart and maintaining low cholesterol levels, the federal government suggests that we get no more than 10 percent of daily fat calories from saturated fat and 10 percent from polyunsaturated fat (visit the web site to view a complete list of daily requirements ⌨). The rest should come from mono-unsaturated fat. I consider this an excellent rule of thumb, but I suggest that you make every effort to concentrate on the monos and polys and keep saturated fat as low as possible. Then you can occasionally afford your favorite meals and restaurant dishes that contain a high amount of saturated fats. I also recommend limiting daily total fat intake to 20 to 25 percent of total calories if you are working to lose a few pounds.

When choosing a fat, lean to the left column and try to avoid the right.

Good Fats	Not-So-Good Fats
Unsaturated	Saturated
Monounsaturated	Hydrogenated oils
Polyunsaturated	Trans-fatty Acids
Omega-3 fatty acids	Cholesterol

Vitamins and Minerals

The popularity and product variety of vitamin and mineral supplements has exploded in the past twenty years. Some researchers, such as Linus Pauling, devoted most of their lives to the study of these chemical structures. There are several new discoveries and claims that focus on particular vitamins and minerals, but most of their actions are simply for sustaining life.

Many products add vitamins and minerals, while others include distilled forms that profess to prolong life or provide immediate energy. The truth to these claims resides in the biochemistry of these important chemicals, and it's simpler than you would think. They are essential for life and exist in all unprocessed foods. Although we are more familiar with vitamins and minerals in a pill, shake, or powder form, these micronutrients naturally come conveniently packaged within our unprocessed protein, carb, and fat macronutrients (if we eat the proper ones).

Many foods we see in grocery stores today are supplemented with "300%" of this particular vitamin, or "50%" of that kind of mineral. Products such as breakfast cereals and bars, waffles, juices, milk, and even some fresh produce now have added micronutrients and thus are labeled "fortified." Unfortunately, many people consume these fortified fruit drinks, veggie chips, milk-like beverages, colorful cereals, and the like, and pat themselves on the back thinking that they are getting all of their necessary micronutrients and more. And although one might argue that a vitamin-enriched sugary soft drink is better than an unfortified one, some foods are low quality no matter how much you supplement them.

MICRONUTRIENT QUALITY VS. QUANTITY

Consider this: unprocessed foods that already have micronutrients in them also have an abundance of additional important chemicals (phytochemicals such as lycopenes, and other antioxidants) that have been shown to help protect you from cancer, heart disease, and other medical conditions. Many of these health-enhancing substances, not to mention the dietary fiber many fruits and vegetables contain, can't be delivered in the same high quality form if placed in a pill or powder.

I consider vitamin and mineral supplementation a personal preference. A lack of any micronutrient is unhealthy, and I do think that supplementation is a good idea in most situations. But some supplements can actually cause problems if taken in high quantities. In general, though, most of the vitamin and mineral products on the market are quite safe and serve as a dietary safeguard when your eating habits fall short of your Dietary Reference Intakes (DRI). If you stick with a product that has close to 100 percent of the DRI for most micronutrients, you can be confident that you aren't "megadosing" yourself—a link to these government standards is also on the web site. 🔖

To help you make more informed decisions, let's take a closer look at what micronutrients really are. These tiny nutrients are actually parts of our metabolic machinery. In biochemistry terms, they are referred to as coenzymes and catalysts. These terms simply describe their function. When acting as catalysts, they help initiate or speed up vital bodily processes; when acting as coenzymes, they are an actual piece of important enzymes, turning them on or making them function better.

Enzymes (especially those that produce vital chemical reactions in your body) require particular vitamins or minerals in order to function properly. Think of one of your enzymes as an automobile. A vitamin or coenzyme is like the car key or the carburetor, and certain catalysts act like high-octane gasoline. You don't have to be a mechanic to know that a shortage of these items might turn your perfectly tuned Ferrari into a sputtering Pinto. Because we cannot synthesize most micronutrients, an absence of certain key vitamins and minerals can slow and even stop certain chemical reactions, causing fatigue, serious health problems, or even death.

So what should you take, how should you take it, and why? These questions can be answered with one word: *bioavailability*. Bioavailability refers to the amount of a substance that your body will recognize, absorb, and utilize.

Remember, our body will not utilize a food or drug well if it is not first recognized or manufactured by your body. And like most drugs and "enhancers," the effects from micronutrients are directly proportional to their ability to work with the normal processes in our bodies.

Whether it's vitamin C from fruits and vegetables, calcium from milk products, or selenium from nuts and seeds, Mother Nature always provides the best brand of vitamins and minerals. If you make the effort to consume good fuels for your machine, you can receive all of the necessary micronutrients from your diet. As changes in your lifestyle occur, you can adjust your eating habits and meal planning.

IRON BIOAVAILABILITY

Iron is a vital part of red blood cells' overall function—their ability to deliver oxygen to our cells. A low intake of this mineral can develop into the medical condition *anemia*. Taking supplements high in iron is a good way to treat this condition, but quite a bit of the iron you get from these supplements is excreted or lost with a visit to the rest room.

The body can absorb iron in supplement form, but it recognizes and readily accepts a more complex natural form of iron completely: hemoglobin. Hemoglobin is a protein molecule that has four specialized "heme" groups that contain iron. Its vital function is to hold on to and release oxygen within our red blood cells, and it is entirely dependent upon iron to do its job. Iron in its hemoglobin form has the highest level of bioavailability. That means beef, poultry, seafood, and eggs deliver close to 100 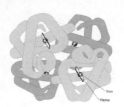 percent of their iron to your body in its hemoglobin form, but don't discount other natural sources such as fruits, nuts, legumes, and vegetables. They might not have the high levels of iron offered in animal products, but they offer a form of iron in their unprocessed state that is also recognized quite easily by our cells.

For example, I eat more vegetables high in calcium and really watch my sodium intake now that I eat more lean protein. If my eating habits temporarily get off-track, depending on the time period, I may take vitamin and mineral supplements. Just keep in mind that taking supplements involves a bit of trial and error. Start with smaller doses (for example, cut a multivitamin in half) or take your supplements two to three times a week at first. Try to begin with vitamin and mineral brands with amounts closer to the DRIs and avoid "megadosing." Also, remember to take supplements with meals. These coenzymes and catalysts need fuel and parts to work with.

Once you've tried this for a few weeks, take the time to evaluate how you feel. Give your body a chance to tell you what it likes, dislikes, and needs. And, as always, any possible health concerns should be directed to your doctor, dietitian, or nutritionist. Thankfully, the benign nature of most common vitamins and minerals in today's market allows a certain experimental freedom if applied in moderation.

Now that you have a solid understanding of the various components of the foods you eat, you're ready to start using the BOK Three Principles of Eating.

BOK Three Principles of Eating

Principle No. 1: How Much to Eat

Who wants seconds? How often have you heard that question at the dinner table? Maybe you come from a family eager to dish out seconds, thirds, or even fourths. Nowhere else on this planet are there more restaurants that promote "All You Can Eat" buffets, "Grand Slam" breakfast meals, or piled-high "Meal Deal" combos that could feed a whole village in a third-world country. Americans demand their food bigger, faster, cheaper, and limitless. This attitude is implanted in our minds at a young age, and it is only getting worse. Childhood obesity is now almost as endemic as adult obesity. We have to destroy this attitude before it destroys us—our health, economy, and way of life.

Eat Less, Live Longer

It is a well-known fact that a high-calorie diet containing too many saturated fats is linked to an increased incidence of heart disease. We also know that a high-calorie diet containing too many carbohydrates, especially the simple (sugary) kind, can sometimes lead to diabetes. Both are life-threatening diseases that can also compromise your quality of life early on and in your golden years. There is now documented scientific evidence that any high-calorie diet can limit your very life expectancy. This evidence first came to scientists' attention during the 1980s when they compared the lifespan of two groups of mice. Each day, one group was given a limitless amount of food and the other group was given 40 percent less than the "all you can eat" group. This was by no means a starvation or even restricted diet; the mice in the limited food group had plenty of food on which to thrive. In fact, the mice that ate less were healthier, had more energy, and lived 20 percent longer than the other group! Translated into human years, that would be on average an extra fifteen quality, healthy years of life. The mice that were allowed to eat at will not only had shorter lives, but also had a higher incidence of diabetes, cancer, and heart disease. They even had less sex! I don't know about you, but this really challenged my view of the old saying "fat and happy." A few human and primate studies, as well as statistics from a few unique cultural groups in other countries, confirm the less food / better health phenomenon. Just like any other machine, if we give our bodies too much fuel and stress our parts beyond their original design, something is either going to break or simply wear out sooner than it should. Watching your caloric intake will not only pay off in your weight management but it will also give you a much better shot at a longer, healthier, and happier life.

Calories to Fit Your Needs

There is no way around it: calories do count. It doesn't matter if you're a low-carb, low-fat, or higher protein kind of eater, in the end it always comes down to how much. To maintain weight and stay fit, how much you eat must be equal to or less than what you burn. This is your highest priority and the reason it is principle number one. But as I promised, you won't have to be a slave to calorie counting. Though some counting is inevitable, especially in the beginning of a new eating program and when making your own meals, I am going to teach you how to make it a quick mental and visual task, rather than a complicated mathematical calculation. And you will still enjoy yourself at mealtime. Taste, frequency, and quality will become your new meal planning priorities. You will not eat less often; you will eat more often. I will show you how eating quality calories within a healthy calorie count will keep you satisfied and burning calories all day long. Now before some of you blow off the first of my three principles as trite or old news, let me clarify its importance. I am not suggesting that you eat like a mouse. Calorie restriction is not my main focus. Eating like a mouse will produce weight loss, but I want you to strike a balance that will be realistic for your lifestyle. Study after study has shown that a diet focused only on calorie restriction is doomed to fail. When people cut calories to lose weight, they eat too little and view it as a temporary sacrifice with the assumption that eating habits will go back to normal once the weight is lost. They are always hungry and miserable, which adds up to an emotional recipe for failure.

I am going to teach you how to figure out your daily caloric needs based on the energy you burn during a day. Then, in Principles 2 and 3, I will show you how to consume the calories you need with an eating style that you can maintain effortlessly.

There are countless ways to determine how many calories you should consume, from charts put out by insurance actuaries and government pamphlets, to sophisticated machines that measure the oxygen you use. I've never been hooked up to a bunch of tubes and dunked in a tank of water, and I am assuming that you don't want to be put through that bother either. You can estimate your daily food intake simply by using your height, age, and gender as factors. Note that I say estimate. You can factor in your activity level or any other personal criteria that can affect the rate at which you burn calories. For example, a waiter in a busy diner will use up more calories than a desk jockey.

The following table provides estimates of total daily calories for thirty-year-old men and women with different heights, weights, and activity levels. The chart was developed by the National Institute of Medicine, a panel of scientists and physicians appointed by the U.S.

Congress to design daily guidelines for adults to maintain a healthy lifestyle. It is not a weight-loss chart, but I like the fact that it provides a range of calories and shows a realistic view of how much the average person can eat daily.

Use these numbers as a starting place and see where your calorie range is. The web site will calculate a more accurate number of calories you burn according to your personal profile. 🔖

Notice that the daily calories for a four feet eleven inches tall sedentary woman and a five feet eleven inches tall active man only differ by a little less than 1,200 calories! It just isn't necessary for a smaller person to eat a lot less or a larger person to eat a lot more to maintain their goals. Rather than focusing on the exact amount of calories you consume, I want you to find a high and low range for yourself and realize just how easy it is to overdo it and how unnecessary it is to under do it.

Keep in mind that these estimates are based on what men and women can eat to maintain their weight. They are not designed for weight loss. If you are overweight, you either are eating more than the chart recommends, are not active enough to burn the necessary calories, or both. By cutting back calories or eating at maintenance levels, any physical activity will automatically help you lose weight until you arrive at the metabolic equilibrium we call your target weight. It may happen slowly, perhaps, but it will happen. This is the healthy way you lose weight and keep it off permanently. At the end of Part 2, I describe two general meal plans. The first is the BOK Fat Loss / Weight Maintenance Meal Plan™, which supports the eating strategy just described. The second is the BOK Accelerated Fat Loss Meal Plan, which is a bit more aggressive, allowing you to achieve results faster, and is only intended for specific shorter-term goals.

NATIONAL INSTITUTE OF MEDICINE DAILY CALORIC REQUIREMENTS

Height Meters (inches)	Activities	Weight for BMI of 18.5 kg (lb)	Weight for BMI of 24.99 kg (lb)	*Energy, Men (kcal/day)		Energy, Women (kcal/day)	
				BMI of 18.5	BMI of 24.99	BMI of 18.5	BMI of 24.99
1.50 (59)	Sedentary	41.6 (92)	56.2 (124)	1,848	2,080	1,625	1,762
	Low Active			2,009	2,267	1,803	1,956
	Active			2,215	2,506	2,025	2,198
	Very Active			2,554	2,898	2,291	2,484
1.65 (65)	Sedentary	50.4 (111)	68.0 (150)	2,068	2,349	1,816	1,982
	Low Active			2,254	2,566	2,016	2,202
	Active			2,490	2,842	2,267	2,477
	Very Active			2,880	3,296	2,567	2,807
1.80 (71)	Sedentary	59.9 (132)	81.0 (178)	2,301	2,635	2,015	2,211
	Low Active			2,513	2,884	2,239	2,549
	Active			2,782	3,200	2,519	2,769
	Very Active			3,225	3,720	2,855	3,141

*For each year below thirty, add 7 kcal/day for women and 10 kcal/day for men. For each year above thirty, subtract 7 kcal/day for women and 10 kcal/day for men.

Matching Fuel Percentages to Your Goals

Now that you have a feel for your healthy range of total daily calories, the next step is to determine a correct mix of carbohydrates, protein, and fat. What are the appropriate portions of these three fuels for fat loss, weight maintenance, or just good health? Even though everyone's daily caloric intake for weight maintenance is a little bit different, all three fuel amounts are determined using the same range of percentages and ratios.

The federal food guidelines issued by the Institute of Medicine of the National Academies, for example, suggest that we get 45 to 55 percent of our daily calories from carbohydrates, 10 to 35 percent from protein, and 20 to 35 percent from fat. This is a far cry from the old recommendations that allowed carbs to reach 70 percent and cut off protein at 15 percent. Bravo, Uncle Sam! Like the DRIs for vitamins and minerals, the federal government issues these numbers as safe and conservative criteria based on the consensus of a panel of experts who use current research to make their recommendations.

> YOU CAN EASILY CUT HUNDREDS OF CALORIES WITHOUT LOSING A BIT OF MEAL SATISFACTION..

The weight maintenance percentages in my plan fall within these ranges, and my accelerated fat loss percentages are only slightly different from the government's recommendations. They are designed to help you lose weight, eat more, and maintain peak health. My protein percentages in the accelerated fat loss plan are 5 percent higher than those suggested by the government (well within the safe range, but far less than popular high-protein diets). Protein has fewer calories than fat per gram, so you can automatically lower the amount of total calories you eat per day by switching to this ratio.

You can easily cut hundreds of calories without losing a bit of meal satisfaction. For example, cutting out just one tablespoon of oil for your salad or a pat of butter for your vegetables saves 110 calories and subtracts nothing from feeling satisfied. Instead, you could consume those same calories by eating three ounces of chicken breast—pure protein that will help satisfy your hunger better and help build fat-burning muscle. Combine that protein with some complex carbs and you have the secret formula for minimizing fat production.

Here are my two suggested sets of fuel percentages and their carbohydrate-to-protein ratios:

BOK FAT LOSS/WEIGHT MAINTENANCE FUEL PERCENTAGES

(Carbohydrate to protein ratio* is 2:1)

Food size percentages in grams:
60% carbohydrates, 30% protein, 10% fat

Food energy percentages in calories:
50% carbohydrates, 25% protein, 25% fat

*You can consume twice as many carbs as protein for both calories and gram weight.

BOK ACCELERATED FAT LOSS FUEL PERCENTAGES

(Carbohydrate to protein ratio* is 1:1)

Food size percentages in grams:
45% carbohydrates, 45% protein, 10% fat

Food energy percentages in calories:
40% carbohydrates, 40% protein, 20% fat

*You can consume the same amount of carbs as protein for both grams and calories.

It's that simple. You can eat twice as many carbohydrates as protein or equal amounts of these two fuels, depending on which plan you choose. As you will learn later in Part 2, the BOK Six Fuel Groups classification system is based on the ratios from the BOK Fat Loss / Weight Maintenance fuel percentages. Note that the percentages are a bit different if you are calculating grams or calories, but either way the carb to protein ratios are the same for each and the only thing I want you to focus on for now.

Please don't feel chained to these percentages. Let's be honest, it is next to impossible to eat exactly by the numbers day in and day out. Once in a while you will forget, miscalculate, or totally fall off the wagon. Ultimately, you should adhere to these guidelines to reach your goals, but they do not need to be perfectly matched at every meal. They only need to add up at the end of the day and total up by week's end. These ratios are a basis for you to develop your own eating habits specific to your own set of goals. I want you to understand them and make them your own, not simply accept them and follow on blind faith alone.

Another benefit of these fuel ratios is their inherent ability to help you navigate different or difficult situations. They work beautifully to quickly adjust a diet gone awry. For example, you can quickly correct the unwanted physical effects of overeating unhealthy foods by returning to your percentages or ratios and recommended calories at your next meal. You don't have to starve yourself the next day if you overindulge; just return to the basics. The same goes for a day when you are fighting fatigue or having a hard time staying focused. Give your body the amount of food it

51

needs, return to a better food percentage scenario, and select better quality fuels before you reach for that double espresso. How about emotional situation that influences your food choices, such as a bad day at work or an argument with a friend or spouse? Returning to the basic principles will put you back on track and avoid a downward spiral.

Just do your best, and before long you'll be keeping a mental log from meal to meal, tallying up the percentages at the end of the day, and you will be able to make intelligent choices quickly.

Sizing Made Simple

If you are looking for a quick and easy visual reference to gauge meal size, just put up your dukes! On average, the inside of your stomach is about the size of your clenched fist after a healthy-sized meal and two fists after a large meal. Think of that next time you approach the all-you-can-eat buffet line at a party or restaurant.

Meal sizes in this country are out of control. We have become big-meal obsessed, mostly as a result of food chains competing among themselves to serve up the "biggest" bang for the buck—most often unhealthy processed carbohydrates and fat. We have to turn this trend around.

So, what is a normal-size serving? The "Simple Serving Size Visual Chart" gives you a visual comparison of what is considered "normal" for a few food items. Think of these visual images each time you sit down at a meal to get a realistic idea of what you need to satisfy that fist-sized stomach. Granted, these might seem meager if you are on the typical three-meal-a-day plan, but they are not on my plans, which encourage you to eat far more than three times a day. The way to lose fat is to eat more often. Principle 2 will explain why and show you how.

> THE INSIDE OF YOUR STOMACH IS ABOUT THE SIZE OF YOUR CLENCHED FIST.

SIMPLE SERVING SIZE VISUAL CHART		
Food	**Serving Amount**	**Visual Image**
Pasta, cooked	1 cup	Size of a baseball or tennis ball
Fruit	1 cup	Size of a baseball or tennis ball
Potato	Medium	Size of a computer mouse
Bagel	2 oz.	Size of a yo-yo
Meat	1 oz.	Size of a matchbox
	3 oz.	Size of a deck of cards, bar of soap, or checkbook
	8 oz.	Size of a small paperback book
Peanut Butter	2 tbs.	Size of a ping pong ball
Nuts	1 oz.	Two shot glasses full
Cottage Cheese, Low/nonfat	1 cup	Size of a baseball or tennis ball
Cheese	1 oz.	Size of four dice

Principle No. 2: How Often to Eat

If you eat the traditional three meals a day but continuously think about food, I have good news for you. You are not eating often enough! Think for a moment. When was the last time you ate? If the answer is four, five, or even six hours ago, you are going way too long between meals. I cannot emphasize this enough: How often you eat is tantamount to reaching and maintaining any weight-loss or weight-management goals. It is the number one workhorse behind the three principles. It is the key to insulin management, a more stable metabolism, and optimal health.

If you want to produce consistent results and avoid the hunger and misery that result from conventional diets, eat smaller portions and eat more frequently—five to seven meals per day. Principle No. 2 makes Principle No. 1 attainable and easy to maintain. Frequent small meals infuse the body with a slow and steady flow of fuels producing wonderful things for the body and mind. Slow and steady keeps insulin and blood sugar levels on an even keel avoiding erratic surges that play havoc with the appetite, dull the brain, and put wear and tear on body systems. Slow and steady keeps the brain (fueled by carbs) continually fed, helping to maintain mental clarity all day long.

Frequent small meals allow us to maintain a higher and more consistent level of protein in the blood, keeping those metabolic engines in our muscles revved up and increasing the rate at which calories are burned. Last, but certainly not least, eating less food more often circumvents hunger and the cravings that accompany it, making life within a healthy caloric limit a slam-dunk. Eating more frequently is the key to a successful weight-loss program because it prevents the typical "sometimes" dieter from quitting. It is also what counts most when it comes to maintaining your hard-earned results. One of the marvels of the body that I mentioned in Part 1 is our ability to store food. It really is incredible, even though most people do not view it as an asset. But think about it: fuel storage is directly related to eating habits for all species. Think of the bear that eats throughout the first three seasons of the year collecting layers of fat. Instead of a burden, the fat storage becomes vital to survival when the bear hibernates without eating all winter. The opposite is true for species like deer or other "grazers." They eat small meals continuously throughout the day and during all the seasons. So if you are unsure about buying into the idea that eating five or six smaller meals a day promotes weight loss, answer this question:

Have you ever seen a fat deer?

Insulin: The Storage Hormone

The main reason small frequent meals are such a successful weight-loss and weight-management tool is because they keep insulin working at a steady pace. And not only will a lower steady level of insulin store less fat, but it will also automatically promote better overall health. Insulin is a life-sustaining hormone that is produced by an organ called the pancreas, where it works as chief liaison to a variety of metabolic events that take place in the body. Primarily, insulin regulates the levels of glucose (sugar) in the blood and is involved in the processes necessary to metabolize, store, and burn carbohydrates, protein, and fat. In short, how insulin acts and re-acts is directly related to our eating habits. And what it reacts to the most is a big meal, especially one containing a lot of carbohydrates.

When we eat a big meal or tease insulin with storage-friendly foods (like simple carbohydrates), the pancreas is pushed into production overdrive, surging the bloodstream with abnormally high levels of insulin. When this happens, the body's fuel-regulating mechanisms run amok. Think of normal insulin secretion as the calm river at the base of the Hoover Dam. What would happen if the dam suddenly broke free? A large meal will break that dam, setting off a tidal wave of insulin causing an overflow of fat storage.

Taking the Glucose-Insulin Ride

In the graph below, the level of glucose (fuel) in the bloodstream peaks about one hour after ingestion and returns to normal levels within a period of two hours for both the three (dashed line) and seven (solid line) meal frequencies. Note that the smaller, frequent meals keep you more in the satisfied range and safer blood sugar levels—larger meals create a cycle of hunger and fullness that promotes unhealthy blood sugar levels.

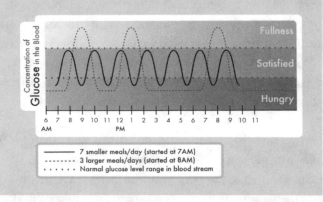

——— 7 smaller meals/day (started at 7AM)
- - - - - - 3 larger meals/days (started at 8AM)
• • • • • • Normal glucose level range in blood stream

The graph below shows the two insulin responses. The seven-meal day (solid line) shows virtually no variation in insulin response and maintains a steady, low level of insulin throughout the day. And since insulin is the storage hormone, the lower the insulin level, the more likely it is that fat will be burned, not produced or stored.

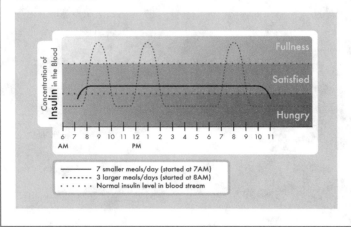

——— 7 smaller meals/day (started at 7AM)
- - - - - - 3 larger meals/days (started at 8AM)
• • • • • • Normal insulin level in blood stream

Insulin is the molecular key that directs carbs, fat, and protein in the blood into the cells where they will either burn as fuel or hibernate in storage. The more we eat, the more insulin is let loose, resulting in greater fuel storage. And if that is not enough to sabotage weight-

> HIGH INSULIN LEVELS…
> WILL BLOCK YOUR
> ABILITY TO BURN FAT AS
> WELL.

loss efforts, high insulin levels hit on fat metabolism directly and will block your ability to burn fat too and bully it back into your fat cells. Give your body more protein and carbohydrates than it can burn and insulin will turn them into fat as well.

The bigger the meal, the larger the release of insulin, and the greater the consequences. Keep that in mind next time you're tempted by thoughts of a high-sugar soft drink and bag of cookies while watching your favorite TV program!

Carbohydrates enter the bloodstream faster than protein and fat because they are the only fuel that is broken down as soon as we start chewing (by an enzyme secreted by the salivary glands). Also, you have learned that carbohydrates are absorbed into the bloodstream at different rates, quality carbs (the complex kind) being the slowest to flow through. However, a large amount of any carbohydrate will create a rush of insulin, so it is in your best interest to eat your carbs smartly so they trickle in slowly. We'll explore this more in our discussion of Principle No. 3.

Principle No. 2 is also important for protein regulation and maintenance. Carbohydrates and fats can be stored in the body and will remain there until they are needed. Protein also has a storage house—our muscles. The difference is that taking protein from storage usually goes against our weight-management goals because it means that we are decreasing muscle mass, which affects our metabolism (this can lower it). Eating small frequent meals with good quality protein will provide a steady supply of this fuel, which is the best and easiest way to maintain a better metabolism and ensure that your body doesn't have to turn to your muscles for the protein it needs to keep burning the other two fuels.

Keep in mind, though, that total daily calories (Principle No. 1) still dominate weight loss and gain. Meal frequency and insulin levels, however, play the lead in our ability to maintain our ideal weight and health because they operate the controls for fat storage. Bottom line: to discourage fat storage, keep insulin at a consistent low level. That means keeping meal frequency a top priority.

How Do I Know When I'm Full?

Another perk of eating frequently is the effect that eating small meals has on the stomach itself. We already know that chemical processes (such as blood sugar and insulin release) are affected by our poor eating habits, but there are mechanical processes that also add to our problems. The stomach walls contain special "stretch receptors" that communicate with the satiety center in the brain, the place where we perceive our sense of satisfaction after a meal or feel discomfort from hunger. As food and beverages make their way down the esophagus, the stomach walls are stretched by the amount that enters. As the stomach stretches, the stretch receptors start sending messages to the satiety center (You can slow down now!). The more food we eat, the stronger the signal and the more satisfied we feel (Enough, already!). However, it takes about twenty minutes for your food signal from the stretch receptors in your stomach to get to the satiety center in your brain. And that's plenty of time for you to wolf down a serious amount of food at any meal.

OVEREATING: THE DOUBLE-EDGED SWORD

There are two common eating habits that send insulin levels into the stratosphere: overeating and eating fat storage–friendly foods, such as large quantities of simple and processed carbohydrates. Notice how the dashed line in the graph below differs sharply from the solid line. Insulin *and* blood sugar rise quickly after the large meal, then take a plunge. This infamous "sugar crash" not only takes the curve lower and makes us hungrier than if we had a small meal, but the strong signal can make you eat again sooner! The result is lethargy, mental fatigue, and even confusion. Unfortunately, the most frequently chosen quick fix is to eat more carbs—something sweet—and that can start a vicious cycle. And now you know the answer to the question: "How could I eat that slice of pumpkin pie after stuffing myself at Thanksgiving dinner?"

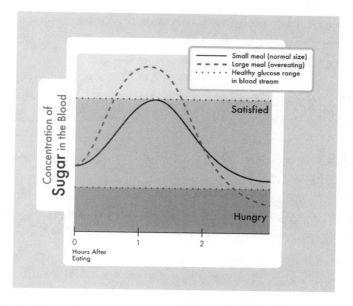

No doubt you've overeaten during the holidays and wondered how you could have eaten so much, right? Well, it's because your brain was operating on a lack of information. While you were enjoying the taste of your meal (a signal that reaches your brain almost instantaneously), your brain was still thinking your stomach was empty. We are able to eat heaping plates of food like ravenous piranhas because the brain doesn't know that the stomach is full yet. Just relax. Eat slowly, chew your food completely, and take short breaks. This way, even the smallest of meals can last longer and give you complete satisfaction.

Gauging portion size is simple if you remember that your stomach is about the size of your fist. And that is the amount of food that it will take to satisfy you. Three-meal-a-day eaters often down the equivalent of two to three fistfuls. It is the feeling of fullness to which they have become accustomed. The stomach can have an average maximum capacity of approximately 1.5 liters—3.5 pounds! Eating large meals only two to three times a day, every day, is a big problem because eventually it stretches the stomach to the point where it stays at its new, larger size. This actually resets the stretch receptors so that they send that full feeling to the satiety center only af-

IT TAKES ABOUT TWENTY MINUTES FOR YOUR FOOD SIGNAL ... TO GET TO YOUR BRAIN.

ter a larger volume of food hits the stomach. As the walls of the stomach are stretched, we become less sensitive to the "fullness" signal. You end up needing more food—more calories—to feel full!

The good news is that for most of us the stomach stretch receptors are very elastic and can snap back over time. Just cut back on your meal size. Eating small, more frequent meals can gradually bring down the stretch threshold and allow the stomach to shrink back to its smallest size, about two ounces (between meals). Your smaller stomach size will guarantee a feeling of satisfaction after a small meal, especially if you allow twenty minutes for meal time, which will allow your brain to register that you've had enough. Be aware, though, that there are other influences on our sense of satiety. For example, did you know that hunger can actually be thirst in disguise? The web site has more about this miscommunication. 📖

Perfecting Timing

Now let's take a look at real-life food requirements, starting with the moment you smack the snooze button on your alarm clock at 6:30 a.m. You yawn, stretch, and rub your stomach, which feels a little empty from your overnight fast. Your body needs energy, though it has probably liberated some of your stored carbohydrates during the night. As a result, you may not feel hungry right away. Sometime within the next half hour to an hour, you feel a little pang. You are ready for your first meal. It should be a small meal because after six to eight hours without food your stomach is at its smallest (and when stretch receptors are most sensitive). You're out the door and on the road a little after 8:00 a.m.

Hopefully, you did not leave home without your morning snack that, calorie-wise, should be about the same size as or slightly larger than your breakfast. You start to nibble on it at about 10:30 a.m. At noon or shortly thereafter, you are ready for lunch. Then at about 3:00 or 4:00 p.m., it is time for food again—just a small snack, about the size of your breakfast or morning snack. At 5:30 p.m., still feeling satisfied from your mid-day snack, you head home to prepare dinner. Calorie-wise it should be close to or slightly less than the size of your lunch. Or, if you were still quite full from your afternoon snack, you may have decided to have a light dinner. If that was the case, two hours before bedtime, at about 9:00 p.m., you may feel hunger returning so you have another small healthy snack or nibble on leftovers from dinner, still being careful not to exceed your total daily calorie requirements. You're off to dreamland right after the 10:00 p.m. news and before you feel your sugar levels drop to avoid the infamous "midnight snack."

PORTION REAPPORTION

Do you habitually eat until you can't eat any more? To break this habit, I suggest you visually and physically divide the meal you are about to eat into four equal parts. Eat each portion at your regular rate and then wait two-to-five minutes before starting on the next portion. Don't, however, just sit there and stare at your food! Converse with a dinner partner, read your mail, page through a magazine or surf the internet. This will give the satiety center in your brain plenty of time to send signals to the stretch receptors in your stomach that you've had enough to eat. Gradually you will feel satisfied eating less food, making it easier to stick with your new eating pace.

Does this measure up to your typical day? If you are reading this book because you want to lose weight, chances are it doesn't measure up at all. Log on to the web site to help you plan your meals and portions. But when it comes to how you vary your calories from meal to meal, do what works best for you. You may, for example, want to have your biggest meal at dinner rather than lunch. Maybe a bigger afternoon snack will help you in the gym after work. You may want to split your dinner in two, substituting the second half for a late snack. Just make sure that your last meal is eaten two hours before bedtime and that your first is within two hours of awakening. The point is to make sure that no one meal is too heavy in calories and that meals are separated by a healthy amount of time.

To illustrate how this measures out, let's use as an example of an active tall woman on a 2,000-calories-a-day diet. She could divide her calories evenly throughout the day (but most of us by nature are not that robotic) or she could vary them, as demonstrated below. Her caloric intake during the day would look like this:

Meal	Five-Meal Plan		Six-Meal Plan	
	Even Calories	Varied Calories	Even Calories	Varied Calories
Breakfast	400	200	330	200
Snack	400	200	330	200
Lunch	400	700	350	700
Snack	400	300	330	200
Dinner	400	600	330	500
Snack	—	—	330	200

See Food, Eat Food

Guess what? Mom was right. Our eyes actually are bigger than our stomachs! In a study at Pennsylvania State University, scientists proved that people eat according to the amount of food on their plates, even though they would be just as satisfied with less. In one of the studies, four teams were offered different size hoagie sandwiches, six, eight, ten, and twelve inches long. The bigger the sandwich, the more they ate. No surprise there! However, those who ate the smallest sandwich reported the same amount of meal satisfaction as those who ate the largest; proof that smaller portions are just as satisfying.

Have I convinced you that small, more frequent meals are the way to go? Good. I cannot emphasize enough how important this step is to your weight-management goals. Equally important is your timing between meals. Remember, the normal rise and fall of both insulin and blood sugar in response to eating is about two hours. As long as you wait at least this amount of time and no more than three hours to eat your next meal, your insulin and blood sugar levels will remain optimal—that is, most consistent—for weight loss and maintenance.

Your life-long mission will now be to eat smaller meals five to seven times a day, about every two to three hours in the typical sixteen-hour waking day. You will eat like this for four important reasons:

1. To avoid the overproduction of insulin and high blood sugar levels

2. To avoid the hunger-promoting "sugar crash," the inevitable drop in blood sugar that occurs when we overeat

3. To enhance the eating experience and avoid hunger pangs
4. To put our body in fat-burning mode and keep it out of fat-storing mode

Next comes the most commonly asked question: what, exactly, is someone supposed to eat in those five to seven meals a day? The answer is the right mix of carbohydrates, protein, and fat to help fine-tune your fat-burning capabilities throughout the day, as described in Principle No. 3.

Principle No. 3: What to Eat

Over the years I have experimented with countless diet plans and different eating habits. I have found that no matter how "revolutionary" or "new" a diet claims to be, you just can't hide from Mother Nature or the basic laws of physics. Mother Nature is a brilliant planner. She has provided us with natural food sources that will not only keep us alive, but make us thrive. Her foods are abundantly rich in the essential nutrients that keep our machines well-maintained and running twenty-four hours a day. It is no coincidence that nearly all the foods that exist in nature contain some amount of the three essential fuels: carbohydrates, protein, or fat. If it were up to Mother Nature, we'd all be lean, mean human machines because we'd eat these fuels instinctively according to her rules! Unfortunately, somewhere in the middle of the twentieth century, an abundance of food production pulled a coup on Mother Nature. It started to infiltrate the country with "well-meaning" innovations such as fast food, all-you-can-eat buffets, he-man helpings, meal deals, and "kids eat free" offers, just to name a few. Common code words started appearing like "processed," "convenience," "prepackaged," and "free refills." Like lemmings, we followed them right to the checkout counter. And by the end of the century, America became the most overfed and fattest nation in the world. It is time to go back and reclaim Mother Nature's good intentions.

The Naked Truth

Although poor food quality and processing are at the heart of our bad eating habits, there are other factors at work. We have also fallen prey to temptation and great advertising. Plus, these unhealthy foods provide ease and convenience that take the edge off a fast-paced life.

Oh, yes, and there is the taste. A lot of this stuff tastes pretty good (you'll find out why as you keep reading). Even the federal government has noticed the errors in our food selection and is trying to steer us back in the right direction. Four times since 1956 the government has issued official government-endorsed food standards. It started by implementing the Basic Four Food Groups, the four equal squares representing grains, meats, dairy, and fruits and vegetables. Progressively, recommendations have changed, now offering the U.S. Department of Agriculture My Pyramid Plan food guide. While it is a useful tool, it does not help us select food according to fuel content. Not all foods in each food group are composed of the same fuels, and they do not have the same physical effects once they enter your body. In short, the present food classification system does nothing to answer the big question: how does one make food choices and plan meals based on the quality and mixture of fuels that can best manage our health and weight?

I created the BOK Six Fuel Groups to help address this problem. It is a dual-action information tool that will help you achieve your weight management goals and attain optimum health at the same time. It measures and breaks down all foods according to their protein, carbohydrate, and fat content to give you a quick read on what kind of fuel you are about to pop into your mouth at mealtime. This classification system is designed to complement the knowledge you have already gained from the quantitative Principles No.1 and No. 2. Principle No.3 is the qualitative fine-tuning that is necessary for permanent weight loss, weight maintenance, optimum health, and productive longevity. It is the same classification system that I developed using my own body as a guinea pig over the years. It took trial and error, but I can tell you (and so can the other people who have used it) that it does exactly what it is designed to do—make you aware of what you put into your body.

BOK Six Fuel Groups

The BOK Six Fuel Groups classification system is designed to focus your food selection on the amount and the ratios of fuels that you eat throughout the day. You already know from Principle No. 1 that the carbohydrate-to-protein ratio for the BOK Fat Loss / Weight Maintenance Meal Plan is 2:1, and for the BOK Accelerated Fat Loss Meal Plan it is 1:1. But how do you keep track of these ratios and exactly what is in the individual foods that you are eating?

The BOK Six Fuel groups will be your guide to making intelligent choices and keeping track of the ratios you choose. The fuel group order does not reflect an absolute hierarchy, although groups 1, 2, and 3 are all lower in fat and group 6 contains most of the unhealthy processed food items. This design not only simplifies your long-term goals, it also makes shopping, cooking, and ordering in restaurants much easier too.

Simply put, weight loss, especially fat loss, is influenced by the mixture and proportions of protein, carbohydrates, and fats, plus the total number of calories eaten each day. You learned about that in Principle No. 1: How Much to Eat. It is also influenced by the size of a meal, the frequency of your meals, and the effect your food selection has on insulin secretion. You learned about that in Principle No. 2: How Often to Eat. Principle No. 3: What to Eat helps the first two work together more efficiently, and the three combined work to produce the best results in a simplistic way. It is so easy, in fact, that before long this knowledge will become second nature.

All foods contain some combination of the three fuels. There are a few foods that contain nearly equal proportions of the three, but most foods are dominant in only one or two fuels. My food classification system uses the BOK Fat Loss / Weight Maintenance Meal Plan percentages (60 percent carbohydrate, 30 percent protein, and 10 percent fat of total grams per food item) as a standard, and then uses the terms *higher* and *lower* to indicate whether the fuels in each food item are above or below those standard percentages. This naturally breaks foods into six unique groups based the amount of carbs, protein, and fat they contain.

BOK Six Fuel Groups

Fuel Groups	Carbohydrates (60% of Total Grams)	Protein (30% of Total Grams)	Fat (10% of Total Grams)
Group 1	Higher	Higher	Lower
Group 2	Lower	Higher	Lower
Group 3	Higher	Lower	Lower
Group 4	Lower	Higher	Higher
Group 5	Lower	Lower	Higher
Group 6	Higher	Lower	Higher

Although the first three groups are lower in fat, there are processed and unprocessed foods in all six groups. For our purposes, processed is defined as any alteration in the natural form of the food item and unprocessed is defined as the unaltered form, but also includes cooked items and pasteurization (dairy products). For example, unprocessed black beans are healthy, but cooking and canning them does not make them unhealthy. Adding salt, fats, and preservatives to the beans during the processing is what makes certain brands less healthy.

*LENTILS, MATURE SEEDS, COOKED, BOILED, WITHOUT SALT (230 CALORIES)

One cup serving contains:
- **58.47** total grams
- **39.86** grams of carbohydrates
- **17.86** grams of protein
- **0.75** grams of fat

The actual gram percentages calculated for each fuel, look like this:

Carb Grams	Protein Grams	Fat Grams
39.86	17.86	0.75
Higher than 60% (or 35.082)	Higher than 30% (or 17.451)	Lower than 10% (or 5.847)

*Group 1: Higher Carbs / Higher Protein / Lower Fat.

*CHICKEN POT PIE, FROZEN ENTRÉE (484 CALORIES)

- **484** total calories or 84.85 total grams
- **42.71** grams of Carbohydrates
- **3.04** grams of protein
- **29.10** grams of fat

Carb Grams	Protein Grams	Fat Grams
42.71	13.04	29.10
Lower than 60% (or 50.92)	Lower than 30% (or 25.455)	Higher than 10% (or 5.847)

*Group 5: Lower Carbs / Lower Protein / Higher Fat

*Values obtained from the USDA Nutrient Database for Standard Reference, Release 18

Breaking down the calories for each individual food would make a book in itself. Check out the BOK Six Fuel Groups interactive program on the web site ⟨▭⟩ or print the entire list of foods to see what types of food are in each of the fuel groups or which fuel group contains one of your favorite foods. It's easy to use, and within each of the BOK Six Fuel Groups you can choose from common food groups (like fruits, beef, vegetables, dairy and egg, soups and sauces, sweets, etc.) that you are more familiar with and then find the individual food items that you like. Once you select a food item, you can select from different serving sizes and see how many grams of carbohydrates, protein, and fat they contain as well as the amount of salt and total calories.

Easy as 1-2-3

Fuel Groups 1, 2, and 3 are the most diet-friendly, simply because they are lower in fat. They should be considered your new comfort foods, meaning that you can feel comfortable eating from these three groups at will as long as you stay within your calorie limits and focus on unprocessed foods. Groups 4 and 5 also have healthy choices, but keep your portions smaller in these two groups and limit the processed varieties. Group 6 contains the foods with the greatest fat-gaining potential. You may or may not choose to completely avoid them, but at least you will know what they are and what they contain.

Don't think for a minute that you will be restricted in your food choices. As long as you stick to the BOK Three Principles of Eating, you will reach your goals eating foods from all six fuel groups. Even if you choose to stay focused and eat foods only from the first three groups, the number and variety of foods is very large—proof perfect of Mother Nature's superb planning skills. Let's take a quick look at the fuel groups and what they offer.

Fuel Group 1
Carbohydrates: Higher
Protein: Higher
Fat: Lower

When looking for low-fat foods that are closer to a 2:1 ratio of carbs to protein, you should focus on Group 1. Eat these at will as long as you are within your calorie count. Group 1 unprocessed foods include, but are not limited to, dairy products, legumes, and vegetables. Consider a typical serving size to be about one half cup for legumes, one half to one cup for vegetables, and six to eight ounces for dairy products.

Fuel Group 2
Carbohydrates: Lower
Protein: Higher
Fat: Lower

Group 2 is where you will find most lean meats, fish, shellfish, and a few dairy products. These are your ideal proteins for weight maintenance because they are lower in fat. This is also the group to turn to when you see your carbohydrate count for the day getting high. Carbs are hard to avoid because they are in so many foods. That's why I love this group; it helps balance the heavy carb days. Return to this group as needed to meet your protein requirements while keeping fat intake low. Common foods in this group are most types of beef, fish, poultry, game meats, egg whites, low-fat or nonfat dairy products, and supplemental varieties of protein (soy and whey). Appropriate serving sizes are three ounces for meat and fish, half a cup for egg whites, eight ounces for low-fat milk or fortified nonfat milk, four ounces for cottage cheese, and one ounce for cheese. If you are following either the 1:1 or 2:1 ratio plan, feel free to eat in this group at will, add carbs thoughtfully, and stay within your daily calorie count.

Fuel Group 3
Carbohydrates: Higher
Protein: Lower
Fat: Lower

Group 3, the high carb family, by far contains the largest food selection. This is where you'll find processed foods like breads, pastas, rice, cereals, crackers, pancakes, and waffles, as well as low-fat and nonfat desserts, such as cakes, cookies, ice cream, and candy. Because these foods are usually higher in simple carbohydrates, you need to approach this group with a little caution. Excess carbs, especially eaten in one sitting, release more insulin, which can turn off the body's fat-burning mechanism and turn on the fat storage—a situation you want to avoid. This means that even though these foods are low in fat, eating a lot of them at once can create a fat-storage friendly environment in your body no matter what you eat with them. The best way to minimize this risk is to opt for unprocessed, complex, quality carbs (such as fruits, vegetables, legumes, and whole grains) or keep your servings smaller and include protein, fat, or other complex carbohydrates in your meals or snacks. Serving sizes in this group are one slice for breads, and one half to one cup for pastas, rice, cereals, fruits, and vegetables.

Fuel Group 4
Carbohydrates: Lower
Protein: Higher
Fat: Higher

This group contains a lot of good protein, but it crosses the line into higher fat percentages. Notice that this group is not just limited to meats. Cheeses, milk, yogurt, and whole eggs have more fat than groups 1 or 2 and more often a higher saturated-to-unsaturated ratio. Soy products have their share of fat, too, though it is unsaturated. Still, when it comes to burning fuel, fat is fat. Plan these foods in your day carefully so that you do not exceed your fat ratio limit. They are not off-limits in any eating program you design; just remember to keep them in the "occasional" category. The caveat "everything is good in moderation" applies here.

Fuel Group 5
Carbohydrates: Lower
Protein: Lower
Fat: Higher

This group is made up of foods that are mostly or purely fat and oils. Nuts, seeds, nut butters, salad dressings, butter, lard, mayonnaise, certain cheeses, a variety of luncheon meats, and oils all fall into this category. Here the serving sizes should never go beyond ounces, teaspoons, or tablespoons. I still believe that nothing should be totally off-limits; however, foods in this group during a weight management plan should be eaten sparingly (somewhere around the suggested 10 percent gram weight and 25 percent calories).

As you know, not all fats are created equal. Fats can be grouped into unsaturated fats (which include monounsaturated and polyunsaturated) and saturated fats. Unsaturated is always the best choice. Monounsaturated fats have shown better protection for heart disease, but other polyunsaturated fats are also very healthy. The foods listed in this fuel group either have two or three types of fat. Almost all plant oils have more mono and polyunsaturated fats, while animal oils are generally higher in saturated fats. For example, olive oil contains more monounsaturated than polyunsaturated than saturated fats.

Fuel Group 6
Carbohydrates: Higher
Protein: Lower
Fat: Higher

A high-fat, high-carbohydrate, low-protein combination is a perfect scenario for fat storage. Such a formula rarely exists in Mother Nature. All of the remaining food items in this fuel category are designed by man, which means many of them are processed and contain additives like salt—another contributor to fat storage. Obviously, this combination constitutes a vast majority of the processed and packaged foods available today. This list could go on and on, but I will keep it simple. Included here are some of the more popular foods, some of which may surprise you. You do not want your fuel mix at the end of the day to add up to this combination, so select these foods sparingly, or not at all

A QUICK WORD ON ALCOHOL

Sugar may be the most abused legalized drug on the planet, but alcohol runs a close second. Not surprising, since both are processed from natural carbohydrates.

There are differences, though, in how the body processes alcohol compared to other carbohydrates. First, alcohol contains seven calories per gram, not four calories per gram like carbohydrates, so it is somewhere between a fat and a carbohydrate in its caloric content. Second, the insulin response is high since most alcoholic beverages (beer, wine, margaritas, etc.) contain simple and other processed carbohydrates with a higher glycemic index. Third, alcohol is the epitome of "empty calories"— totally devoid of any vitamins, minerals, or nutritional value. It contributes no health value to the body, so it quite literally sloshes around in your bloodstream while it does funny things to your brain that can promote fat storage. Drinking alcohol and eating improperly often go hand in hand—the perfect scenario for fat production.

Even just a few drinks will culminate in a sugar crash, which will quite often lead to a late-night binge. And this brings us to the final negative effect: alcohol's effect on the central nervous system. You don't have to get rip-roaring drunk to initiate this problem; you can just sip your way to what is called "disinhibition."

Once you have a drink or two, logical thinking can become clouded. Disinhibition and alcohol sugar are a powerful combination that will work against your goals. Once you have disinhibited your intelligent, healthy, good intentions with enough alcohol, your primitive instincts take over—the ones that tell you to eat like there is no tomorrow.

On the other hand, recent research supports the idea that one to two glasses of wine a day promotes good cardiovascular health. At an average of 100 calories per glass, this moderate amount should not affect your weight. However, keep alcohol in the occasional category if you are on the BOK Fat Loss / Weight Maintenance Meal Plan, and try to avoid it as much as possible if you are on the BOK Accelerated Weight Loss Meal Plan.

The Fat Cocktail

What do you get when you mix sugar, salt, and fat?

Answer: a cocktail that promotes fat production and storage!

If you really want to sabotage your weight-loss and weight-maintenance efforts, just make sure that your meals contain simple carbohydrates, salt, and fat. Eating the three together is like mixing gin, beer, and wine during a night on the town. The combination does far more damage than any one alone, and a fat hangover lasts much longer than an alcohol hangover. While fat by itself is an obvious waist expander, adding salt and sugar will increase the release of the storage hormone insulin. And consuming a Fat Cocktail™, like having one drink, can leave you wanting more.

Here's why: The pure sugar found in foods like candy, cake, and doughnuts gives your body a 100 percent shot of simple carbohydrates. Unlike complex carbohydrates (the kind we get from vegetables and some fruits) that trickle into the bloodstream, simple carbs make a mad dash through your body, kicking insulin into overdrive. To add insult to insulin, most of the processed products that contain the simple carbs also contain *salt* or *sodium*. When salt and sugar enter your system together, they turn on a specialized protein in the intestines that literally *pumps* more sugar into the bloodstream, even if your bloodstream contains as much sugar as it can normally handle from a large meal or sweet dessert. When this happens, the body responds as if you ate more carbs than you really did and releases more insulin. This means everything you ate—not just the sugar and salt, but also the extra protein, fat, and other carbs—will be more easily stored as fat.

Remember that a high level of insulin also temporarily disables the body's fat-burning capabilities. In biochemical terms, the high levels of insulin being forced into the bloodstream shut down the very enzyme that works to break down fat so the body can burn it. In the end, the fat from your meal or any extra calories still hanging around from an earlier meal are then easily escorted into your fat cells. The result: fat storage is maximized—the perfect Fat Cocktail!

> SALT AND SUGAR...TURN ON A SPECIALIZED PROTEIN...THAT LITERALLY *PUMPS* MORE SUGAR INTO THE BLOODSTREAM.

The Fat Cocktail Is Everywhere

Unfortunately, you don't have to show your ID if you want the Fat Cocktail. Anyone can get it anytime they want. The Fat Cocktail is available in many forms including all the snacks and processed foods found on grocery store shelves. Desserts are the main offenders but other manufactured food can yield the same chemical makeup. Potato chips, crackers, white bread, breakfast cereals, frozen dinners, cheese puffs, doughnuts, cookies, cakes, brownies, candy, chocolate bars, and ice cream make up some of the more popular Fat Cocktails. Just a few over-indulgences during the week can negate your weight loss efforts or even worse add a few more unhealthy pounds. The body is simply not built to process foods that counter Mother Nature's design. This is why there are only a few natural foods that contain the combination of high fat, carbohydrates, and salt. Whole milk, for example (has fat, carbs, and a little

> SUGAR + SALT + FAT = MORE FAT PRODUCTION + NO FAT BURNING = MORE FAT STORAGE

sodium), is designed for young mammals to gain weight during periods of growth and development. High-fat, high-carbohydrate foods, a predominately man-made design, constitute the foods found in Group 6 of the BOK Six Fuel Groups. These are the foods you should watch out for—not only because of the way they store fat, but also because of the sluggish way they make you feel, both physically and mentally.

The combination of fat and carbohydrate creates the perfect fat-gain environment. Pour on the salt and you've put fat storage in high gear. The BOK web site has a great diagram that shows how those pumps in your intestine turn the sugar-salt combination into a Fat Cocktail. 📖

The Taste Cover-up

Foods high in fat, and/or high in sugar and added salt, account for many of the processed items that we purchase at the supermarket. Why? Because combining these ingredients in one product may double or even triple its profit potential. The combination creates this demand because of how it affects your taste buds. There is an interesting phenomenon that occurs when we mix sugar and fat. Both make their presence known, but both decrease the sensation we receive from the other. The sugar covers up the fat sensation, and vice versa. The combination of sugar and fat tend to lessen the effect of each and cause you to eat more than if they were eaten separately. The same goes for salt. Salt can also cover up a sugary taste, and sugar can mask higher levels of salt.

> SODIUM ONLY COMES PACKAGED NATURALLY IN ANIMAL PRODUCTS; PLANTS DO NOT HAVE THE ABILITY TO MAKE IT.

All three items hang out in the Fat Cocktail, and they also do a good job of hiding out. For example, you can taste the sugar in ice cream, cookies, and even some granola bars, but can you taste the salt? Probably not, because the taste is overpowered by the other two ingredients. Once I found out about this phenomenon, I made the connection with my children on trips we used to take to the ice cream store. I never understood why my girls would cry out for water after they polished off their ice cream cones. I finally realized the salt was making them thirsty!

Remember that sodium only comes packaged naturally in animal products; plants do not have the ability to make it (just like cholesterol). Check out the sodium content in some of the processed food items that you like to eat and you will be surprised that almost all contain some salt. And that is the biggest challenge with Principle 3. We usually choose What to Eat by the way it tastes. Principles 1 and 2 may be easy to understand on paper and truly work the best for your weight management, but we still have to choose the foods that support these principles. Taste, in reality, is the only obstacle between eating the "right" and "wrong" foods for health and weight management. As we discussed above, it's a powerful obstacle because it is literally "wired" to our survival instincts. We simply need to use a different wiring system to switch from our lower brain to our higher brain. Instead of sugar and salt driving our choices for food, choosing to eat healthy foods can actually change those taste preferences. For example a tuna melt sandwich is tuna mixed with mayonnaise and grilled between two slices of bread with added cheese. Choosing to switch to tuna mixed with low-fat yogurt on whole grain bread or into red bell pepper halves with some seasoning, not only removes the fat, salt, and simple carbs, but adds fiber, vitamins, and minerals. Although I admit that the taste is different, it is quite good even using the old survival taste instincts. Now add to that the fact that with every savory bite you are fighting disease, fortifying your health, maintaining your weight, as well as prolonging your life, and that meal could be one of the best things you have ever tasted. Before long your old survival instincts as well as emotions attached to comfort foods will be replaced with a new wellness instinct and healthy relationship with food.

WHY WE CRAVE SUGAR AND SALT

Our taste for sugar and salt is inherited from our ancestors, who needed them to survive because they do such a great job at helping the body accumulate calories and store fat. To ensure that this instinct remained intact, we were wired with a mechanism to sense their presence—the tongue.

The salt and sugar taste buds are concentrated right up front to better greet these substances as soon as you open your mouth. The signal they send goes directly to one of the most primitive centers of our brain stem and causes a positive response to eat and want more. The brain stem says, "Mmm, good. Me no starve."

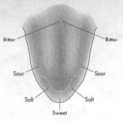

Sour and bitter, which most of us have been programmed to be less interested in, are located on the sides and the back of the tongue.

The Truth Behind the Labels

In my opinion, food from Mother Nature should be the main staple in everyone's diet, no matter how much or how often they eat, no matter how slim or heavy they are, no matter if they are vegetarians or meat eaters. Mother Nature provided all of the nutrients to build and fuel the ideal human specimen way back when, so why do we continue to mess with a great thing by replacing them with processed foods? I believe we all have good intentions but convenience, busy lifestyles, and temptation all get in the way of healthy eating. And then there are the miscues we're given when we load up our carts at the grocery store. So many of us rely on food labels as we shop, but do they provide all of the information we need? Or do we really understand all of it? I am not suggesting that food labeling laws are designed to hoodwink us, but without a degree in nutrition, some ingredients are at best confusing and at worst misleading. Though most of the information on labels is straightforward, you often need to read between the lines to avoid some common misinterpretations.

As for me, label reading has forever changed the way I shop in the grocery store. Food shopping used to be a ten-minute no-brainer, back when my top priorities were ease of preparation and cost control. A frozen pepperoni pizza, a package of hot dogs, a couple cans of creamed corn, and off to the check-out line I went. When I began my healthy crusade, I started to read nutrition labels randomly while shopping. My newfound knowledge dramatically changed my shopping experience. I eventually examined every package, box, can, bag, or jar I considered purchasing. So many items are off my shopping list as a result of label reading that I now skip entire aisles in the grocery store. A patient at one of my clinics once asked, "So where are most of the foods that we should avoid at the store, Doc?" Because healthy, unprocessed foods are commonly found at the perimeter of most markets, I replied, "Almost everything in the middle."

Reading labels may feel like a chore at first, but trust me, the education you'll get and the discoveries you'll make regarding your own eating habits will be time well spent. Before long, you will be dashing through the market, stopping only now and again to take a quick peek at the back labels of a few new items that catch your eye.

Interpreting the Nutritional Facts

Nutritional information on product labels is regulated by the federal government, so label formats look pretty much the same from item to item. Let's take a look at a can of refried beans (no salt added).

There are two sections of every label: Nutrition Facts and Ingredients. Your ability to figure out and evaluate what these two sections are telling you about the amounts and types of carbohydrates, proteins, fats, vitamins, and minerals a packaged food product contains is essential for your healthy diet and weight maintenance success. But before you skip right to these numbers, there are two values you need

REFRIED BEANS

Nutrition Facts

Serving Size !/2 cup (129g)
Servings Per Container about 3 1/2

Amount Per Serving	
Calories 100	Calories from Fat 0
	% **Daily Value***
Total Fat 0g	0%
Saturated Fat 0g	0%
Cholesterol 0mg	0%
Sodium 0mg	0%
Total Carbohydrate 19g	6%
Dietary Fiber 6g	24%
Sugars	2g
Protein 5g	10%
Vitamin A 0%	Vitamin C 0%
Calcium 4%	Iron 6%

*Percent Daily Values are based on a 2,000 calorie diet.

INGREDIENTS: WATER, PINTO BEANS, SUGAR, VINEGAR, CALCIUM DISODIUM EDTA (To Promote Color Retention), GARLIC POWDER, GREEN BELL PEPPER, and SPICE. NOT A SODIUM FREE FOOD to check first: "Serving Size" and "Servings per Container," which are always listed first and in fine print. The only items in the Nutritional Facts that are in **bold** print are the **Amount Per Serving**, **Calories**, **% Daily Values**, **Total Fat**, **Cholesterol**, **Sodium**, **Total Carbohydrate**, and **Protein**.

Notice that these bolded values are *per serving*. One of the biggest mistakes consumers make is assuming that the grams and calories that are listed are calculated for the entire package, can, bag, or box (probably because our appetites are conditioned to see it them as a serving for one person). For example, according to this label, the can of refried beans contains 3½ servings (about 129 grams each). So the calories listed on the label that correspond with the list of values in the nutritional information is not what we are actually holding in our hand—350 calories of refried beans. To figure out the nutritional values of the whole container (since we usually do not eat the exact serving size suggested on the label), you must multiply each value by 3.5, then divide the total by the number of servings you really intend to dish out. That's not simple arithmetic when you are standing in the middle of a food aisle.

Just keep in mind that serving sizes vary for similar products. Most manufacturers utilize the standard, accepted serving sizes for particular food items or food groups though (one tablespoon of ketchup, one ounce of nuts, one cup of soup, etc.). The fractionated number of total servings is usually a result of the container size they have chosen and is usually unintentional.

SUPPLEMENT BARS—MORE THAN YOU BARGAINED FOR

Food supplement bars, meal replacement bars, sport bars, and protein bars are notorious for confusing the consumer. The calorie amount and ingredient percentages (listed in bold print) may look pleasing until you notice that the little bar is more than one serving (listed in fine print)! Why? My guess is that a product with 200 calories per serving and two servings sounds and looks a lot better to the customer than 400 calories per serving and one serving.

Can you see how a quick glance at the calorie count on a label can be misleading if you don't carefully compare serving size, and ingredients before making your purchase? The government mandates that packages must have nutrition labeling, but it is up to manufacturers to set their serving sizes. Hopefully, in the future, there will be standards set for all serving sizes, but for now, it's your job to keep an eye on those labels.

Hidden Information

Label confusion, however, does not end there. There are other important hidden facts that can be both helpful and harmful to your health and weight-management goals. For example, the total carbohydrates listed will not always be the amount available to burn as energy. If the food contains indigestible (insoluble) fiber, the fiber value should be subtracted from the total carbohydrate value since not all of the fiber can be burned as fuel.

Furthermore, there are a few substances that are used by the body but are not yet a part of the government requirements for label listing, such as *glycerine* (four calories per gram). So when the total calories don't equal the amount of carbs, protein, and fat (calculated from their respective calories per gram), you will know that there is something in the Ingredients not calculated into the Nutrition Facts. Go to the web site if you would like to see how to find these hidden calories on your own.

A quick look at the process by which food manufacturers calculate the amount of carbs, fat, and protein will clear up a couple other labeling mysteries. The total carbohydrate value is actually a subtracted, indirect value which results in calories "left over" after protein and fat calories have been calculated. There are better ways to test each product for the exact amounts of protein and fat (the testing is done at the food manufacturer's expense). These specific tests are performed for fat, protein, and total calories only. In some cases the total calories are calculated by

THE FDA DEFINES... SUGAR... AS "THE SUM OF ALL FREE MONO- AND DISACCHARIDES."

burning the product and calculating the heat given off. The total calorie value minus calories calculated from fat and protein equals the total carbohydrate calorie value. And that includes anything "extra" from the packaging process minus the ash from the heat testing process.

On the positive side, the USDA has given "total carbohydrate" a subset for the amount of "sugars." So now it is easier to identify them in the ingredients portion of a label and limit the number of insulin-stimulating simple carbs in your diet.

Interpreting Ingredients

Ingredients are listed by weight, beginning with the largest item and ending with the smallest. Many products can be ruled in or out of your diet simply by checking the first three to five ingredients. Packaged foods usually contain food dyes and thickening agents in order to give food consistency, eye appeal and shelf life. These added ingredients are a fact of life if you are going to eat packaged or processed foods, but thankfully they are in small doses.

For the sake of a healthy diet, you need to check for key words with hidden meanings that can sabotage your diet. Because most products with labels are processed, the main offenders to watch out for are processed carbohydrates. Foremost is the key word *enriched* because it means that most of these foods have been stripped of their natural vitamins and minerals and processed into behaving more like a simple carbohydrate. Commercial grade flour is obtained by removing the germ, fiber, and nutrients from wheat or other grains. In order to give it a nutritional boost, manufacturers have to put something back into it, enabling them to make the claim, "enriched with important vitamins and minerals."

Some other ingredients sound harmless but are really wolves in sheep's clothing, hiding behind common or complex chemical names. For example, canned fruit contains its natural fructose but it can also contain added high fructose corn syrup (HFCS) which is concentrated simple carbohydrates. HFCS is only partially fructose; the rest is processed sucrose or table sugar! Another example is maltodextrin, which is an easily digestible starch similar to modified food starch. Mannitol and sorbitol are alcohol sugars. All can contribute to an unnatural response to food and eventually more fat storage.

The word *hydrogenated* describes a type of oil or fat. Hydrogenating any unsaturated fat or oil (sunflower, safflower, corn, soybean, etc.) automatically turns it into a saturated fat. Any product listing hydrogenated oil high in the ingredient ranking should be on your "nix it" list.

More importantly, hydrogenation produces a type of unhealthy saturated fat called *trans fat* that is not made by Mother Nature. Trans fat is the worst kind of fat because it not only clogs arteries and can contribute to heart disease; it can directly damage your cells.

Bottom line: Be cautious if any undesired ingredient is placed at the beginning of the Ingredient line-up. However, you needn't be too concerned about ingredients less than 1 gram or those proceeded by "contains less than 2% of the following items."

> HYDROGENATING ANY FAT OR OIL AUTOMATICALLY TURNS IT INTO A SATURATED FAT... MORE IMPORTANTLY... UNHEALTHY... *TRANS FAT.*

Some manufacturers already do include more information on their labels than is required by government regulations. Hopefully, this will eventually become the norm.

And that brings me back to the point I made at the beginning of this section. If we'd just stick with Mother Nature and concentrate our shopping in the fresh produce aisles, we wouldn't have to wonder about what we are really putting in our bodies. When it comes to Mother Nature's products, what you see is what you get.

WOLVES IN SHEEP'S CLOTHING

A lot of ingredients found in packaged foods either sound harmless or are disguised by complex or chemical names that require scientific translation. This goes for both friendly and unfriendly weight-management items. In addition, the list of all possible ingredients is huge. The following is a list of some of the more common ingredients that you should look out for, particularly if they appear at the beginning of the list of ingredients.

Ingredient Facts
- **Enriched flour** – Processed grain stripped of its natural micronutrients and fiber; has a higher GI index.
- **High fructose syrup** – Contains processed fructose and sucrose with higher GI than natural fructose
- **Modified food starch** – Thickening agent that is primarily processed carbs with a higher GI
- **Maltodextrin** – Another polysaccharide that is primarily processed carbs with a higher GI
- **Monosodium glutamate (MSG)** – Taste enhancer that adds more sodium to your diet and can cause headaches
- **Glycerine** – Part of a fat molecule that has four calories per gram and is not counted in the Nutrition Facts
- **Hydrogenated oils** – Conversion of unsaturated oils to saturated fat produces trans-fatty acids
- **Lard** – Fat from animal sources with a very high level of saturated fat

Nothing's Free in Life

I don't want to go on a rant here, but if the Fat Cocktail that suffuses our American eating habits isn't bad enough, our food manufacturers made matters worse by trying to "help." A whole slew of products hit the shelves in the 1980s specifically targeting people who wanted to lose weight. They removed the fat and replaced it with, among other things, more sugar and salt.

Some "fat-free" products are still on the shelves today—all with weight-loss slogans and good-for-you innuendos. Again, we're dealing with a double-edged sword. Yes, manufacturers have been successful at extracting the fat from such items as cookies, crackers, cakes, and even TV dinners without losing all of the texture and flavor.

The intention may have been a good one, and the products could be nice treats for consumers if they approached them cautiously to satisfy an occasional craving or to enhance an otherwise nutritious snack. But this isn't what usually happens. For the most part, the fat-free logo acted as a hall pass for bingeing or became the focus of an obviously misguided weight-loss program. Whether its cookies, crackers, potato chips, cereals, prepared meals, or vitamin-enriched meal replacement bars, the large portions once ingested during an occasional overindulgence have been replaced with "guilt-free" inhalation of the whole package, box, tub, or bag—all without a speck of fat! What a deal!

Well, here's the real deal. When manufacturers take fat out, they have to put something back in to satisfy our taste buds. It is usually sugar, high fructose corn syrup, concentrated fruit juices, maltodextrin, or alcohol sugars; these are usually accompanied by enriched flour products, modified food starch, and added salt. It may be fat-free sitting on the plate, but it will become fat in your body if you provoke insulin with the dangerous sodium and simple carb duo. In the end, you'd be much better off eating an ordinary portion of a particular snack's fat-containing and/or lower-sodium counterpart.

Don't get me wrong. This is not finger-wagging time. I too have fallen prey to the no-fat, low-fat temptation. I've been known to inhale an entire family-size bag of salty, baked, low-fat tortilla chips while watching a football game. And I've paid the price. I usually wake up after halftime with my cheek stuck to the couch in a puddle of drool ready to tear into another bag. Hell hath no fury like a pancreas scorned! But this was

FAT FREE CHOCOLATE CHIP COOKIES

Nutrition Facts

Serving Size 1 cookie (16g)
Servings Per Container about 12

Amount Per Serving

Calories 50	Calories from Fat 0
	% Daily Value*
Total Fat 0g	0%
Saturated Fat 0g	0%
Cholesterol 0mg	0%
Sodium 30 mg	1%
Total Carbohydrate 12g	4%
Dietary Fiber 0g	0%
Sugars 7g	
Protein 1g	10%
Vitamin A 0%	Vitamin C 0%
Calcium 0%	Iron 2%

*Percent Daily Values are based on a 2,000 calorie diet. Your daily values may be higher or lower depending on your calorie needs.

INGREDIENTS: Sugar, enriched flour (wheat flour, niacin, reduced iron, thiamine mononitrate [vitamin B1], riboflavin [vitamin B2], folic acid), skim milk, corn syrup, fructose, cocoa* (processed with alkali), chocolate*, soy lecithin* (emulsifier), modified food starch, baking soda, corn starch, salt, potassium sorbate added to preserve freshness, artificial flavor. *Adds a back in the days when I was unaware of what I was doing to my body. You too may have been as clueless as I was then. But now you know that the fat-free trend is no free ride. Getting fat-free products to work for, instead of against, your weight-loss goals requires just two things: realistic portion control and insightful label reading.

Let's take a look at the label on one of the more popular fat-free confections that flew off the shelves when first introduced—fat-free chocolate chip cookies.

The nutritional facts on this label make this fat-free snack look pretty good—until you really look closely at the ingredients. The first two ingredients listed are sugar and enriched flour, and corn syrup, fructose, and modified food starch are also quite high in the lineup. Five major ingredients are processed carbs! And all are high glycemic index carbohydrates, typical for this type of product. It almost doesn't matter which ingredient comes first, since they combine to release more insulin than foods containing more natural carbs. But hey, it's just one little cookie, right? Unfortunately, we know that it would be easy for five or ten of those neat, tasty little snacks to disappear from the box in one sitting. Do the math: 5 to 10 little cookies are 250 to 500 calories and 150 to 300 mg of sodium.

Other Popular Label Claims
So how do all of the claims on food labels get monitored, and by whom? Fortunately, the government has issued guidelines as to what manufacturers can claim when declaring a food "low," "light," or "free" of any item. But again, there is room for deception, since the claims are made on a "per serving" basis. This means that a food that is too high in certain ingredients to qualify as "lite" at a cup per serving could qualify if the serving size is reduced to one-half cup. So you must use your math skills and check the Nutritional Facts, regardless of what the front of the package claims.

Following are some of the guidelines for manufacturing claims as defined by the U.S. Food and Drug Administration:

Manufacturing Claim	Government Definition
Calorie Free	Fewer than 5 calories per serving
Low Calorie	40 calories or fewer per serving
Light or Lite	1/3 fewer calories or 50% less fat per serving than regular brand
Fat Free	Less than 1 gram of fat per serving
Low Fat	3 grams of fat or less per serving
Sodium Free	Less than 5 milligrams per serving
Very Low Sodium	35 milligrams or fewer per serving
Low Sodium	140 milligrams of sodium or less per serving
High Fiber	5 grams of fiber or more per serving
Cholesterol Free	Less than 2 milligrams of cholesterol per serving and 2 grams of saturated fat or less per serving
Low Cholesterol	20 milligrams of cholesterol or less per serving and 2 grams of saturated fat or less per serving

There are other fat-free and low-fat foods that seem like they are very healthy for you, even ones high in protein (lunchmeats, prepared meals, etc.). Read their labels and you will find that they have different amounts and types of added simple carbohydrates and a lot of salt. In addition a whole new variety of low-sugar and sugar-free products have entered the market since the introduction of the "low carb" craze that are not always as "low" or "free" as you are led to believe. Go the web site [📖] and check out the Fat-Free Turkey Chili and Sugar-Free Chocolate Chip Cookie labels to see what I am talking about. The ingredients and their amounts will surprise you.

Am I saying that all processed food items with special dietary claims are off limits? Certainly not. Just prioritize your goals, apply them to your BOK Three Principles of Eating, and see how much of this stuff you can realistically afford to eat and still reach your goals.

With a little investigation, you may find that some of your old favorites or other products you were avoiding actually may have better label profiles. A little extra time spent reading labels will help you stick to Principle No. 3 so you can get the results you want without totally giving up the lifestyle you enjoy.

Next we have combined what you have learned here with the other two principles to develop two eating plans that you can choose from or use to create your own personalized meal plan.

Two Eating Plans to Reach Your Goals

In a perfect world, we would be "one size fits all" human machines. Happy and energized, we would move through work, leisure, exercise, and everyday life situations in perfect stride. Our "engines" would burn exactly what we consume each day, and we would have the same results from any diet and exercise plan we tried.

Now, let's get back to the real world, the one in which we all struggle just to maintain our individual machines. Stop and think about it: you are a unique individual. And because of that, not all prepackaged diets and fitness plans can possibly work for you. While we all share a common goal of optimal health and fitness, because we are unique in our thinking, physical makeup, and fitness goals, we must follow different paths on our journeys. What works for you may not work for me, and that's precisely what is wrong with the cookie-cutter diets so pervasive in today's culture.

I've never liked the word diet because it conjures up images of deprivation, a short-term, unnatural state of existence. But the dictionary definition of diet is: the usual food and drink of a person or animal. That's how I would like you to think of the word diet from now on. Your Body of Knowledge program will include your own personalized eating plan that will become second nature to you. As with anything you have to learn, like a foreign language or a particular skill, you have to think about it at first, try it out, and then it becomes a part of you, like riding a bicycle. You will naturally adhere to a particular way of eating and exercising because initially you will feel better and look better. Quite possibly for the first time in your life, you will enjoy eating in a way that is natural to your daily routine, from the time you wake up until the time you go to bed. For example, are you starving as soon as you wake up in the morning? Then, that is when you'll have your first meal. Can't stand the thought of food first thing in the morning? Then you'll wait an hour or so before you eat. Is lunch your favorite meal of the day, or is it dinner? Whichever, you will eat your "big meal" according to your preference.

There are only three suggestions I have if you truly want to manage your weight and attain optimal health:

1. Stay close to your daily target calories and optimal fuel proportions.
2. Eat five to seven times a day—that is, less food more often.
3. Eat more unprocessed foods and minimize the processed items, and added salt.

I developed my two primary BOK meal plans, for Fat Loss / Weight Maintenance and Accelerated Fat Loss, to help you achieve that ideal weight, peak energy level, and optimum health.

If you are at your ideal weight now, the BOK Fat Loss / Weight Management Meal Plan will allow you to maintain your results easily. If you are overweight now, this plan will help you lose fat and weight, gradually and healthily, until you reach your goals. Then without changing a thing, you will be able to manage your weight and fitness with the same plan. Fat loss may come slowly at first, but it will come without starvation or ridiculous restrictions. You will naturally eat your way to your new healthy weight.

If you want to lose fat at a faster, but still safe pace, you can follow the BOK Accelerated Fat Loss Meal Plan. Depending on your current weight, you could lose pounds and fat faster in the first month and continue to lose each month until you hit your healthy target weight. At that point you can switch to the BOK Fat Loss / Weight Maintenance Meal Plan, which will enable you to remain at your healthy weight.

Both plans will teach you to properly balance your carbohydrate and protein intake, make healthier food choices, and choose better serving sizes. The food item or meal percentages are generally expressed in terms of calories by government recommendations and scientific studies, but you will be making most of your decisions based upon grams or weight.

CALORIES VS. GRAMS

Depending on whether you are counting grams (amount of food) or calories (for your energy intake), there is some variation in the protein to carbohydrate ratios I propose in my dietary plans. Evaluating gram percentages is the easiest way to track your fuel intake and is the reason the BOK Six Fuel Groups food classification system is based on gram percentages and works so well to help you make food choices.

Here are two general rules to follow:
1. Use gram/weight fuel percentages for cooking at home, eating in restaurants, when reading labels, when you are on the go and food size is your only cue.
2. Use calorie/energy fuel percentages when calculating your daily or weekly calorie intake and when comparing government and industry standards.

Use the gram percentages when weighing food and adding up grams on food labels, but use the ratios when ordering meals or any place where they are prepared according to other standards. Whether it is a frozen dinner, a bowl of cereal, or a pita pocket filled with tuna salad from a restaurant, weight directly correspond to the *size* of the portion. For example, don't think that eating within the BOK Fat Loss / Weight Maintenance percentages means that 25 percent of the food on your plate can be fat. That 25 percent refers to calorie values which cannot be visualized, but the 10 percent refers to the size (grams) or amount of fat you can see on your plate or on a food label. This simply shows that the butter, oils, or other fat products in your meal should visually be about one-tenth of the food on your plate, not a quarter.

Grams or weight of your food is what you actually *see* on your plate, which will make your carb and protein calculations even easier. For example, if you follow the BOK Accelerated Fat Loss Meal Plan (1:1 carb-to-protein ratio), make sure that the amount of chicken breast (protein) you are eating is about the same amount as your portion of brown rice and broccoli (carbs). Similarly, if you are following the BOK Fat Loss / Weight Maintenance Meal Plan (2:1 carb-to-protein ratio), make sure that your meatballs (protein) are at least half the amount of the spaghetti (carbs) on the plate.

If this is enough math for you and you feel good about making these decisions on your own, then I have done my job. But if you are a science geek like me and want to know the details, the web site offers a full explanation in "Grams and Calorie Conversions."

BOK Fat Loss/Weight Maintenance Meal Plan

Principle No. 1: How Much to Eat

If you haven't done so already, go to the web site, register, and enter your profile information (height, weight, age, gender) to calculate your daily calories with the BOK Activity and Exercise Planner. Be honest about your activity level. An office worker is probably not as active as a sales clerk in a busy department store or a construction worker.

Your fuel percentages and ratios are as follows:

BOK FAT LOSS/WEIGHT MAINTENANCE FUEL PERCENTAGES

(Carbohydrate to protein ratio* is 2:1)

Food size percentages in grams:
60% carbohydrates, 30% protein, 10% fat

Food energy percentages in calories:
50% carbohydrates, 25% protein, 25% fat

*Remember that you can consume twice as many carbs as protein for both calories and gram weight.

Principle No. 2: How Often to Eat

There are two possible approaches to determining how many calories you should consume each time you eat. With the agreement that you should be eating a minimum of five times a day, logically you would divide your calories equally among your meals. For example, 2,000 calories divided by five meals is 400 calories per meal. Eating the same number of calories every two and a half to three hours is the ideal way to keep your insulin levels steady.

Most people, however, prefer to have a "bigger meal" or two during the day. Not only does this follow old traditions, but these meals may also be necessary to fuel your body at certain times of the day when you are burning more energy. Depending upon your workload or exercise schedule, lunch, dinner, or your late snack can be larger than your breakfast and early snack, or vice versa. The rule of thumb is that the caloric value of your largest meal should not be more than twice the value of your calories if they are split evenly. For example, an even distribution of a 2,000 calorie-a-day plan is 400 calories per meal. Therefore, the largest meal of the day should be no bigger than 800 calories.

Your meal times should fit into your individual lifestyle. However, you should wait a minimum of one and a half hours before your next meal, and do not go longer than three hours between meals.

SAMPLE BOK FAT LOSS / WEIGHT MAINTENANCE DAILY MENU (BASED ON 2,000 CALORIES A DAY)			
Meal	Even Calories	Suggested Calories	Food Examples (for Suggested Calories)
Breakfast	400	200	1 poached egg, 1 orange, 1 slice of toast with dab of butter
Morning Snack	400	200	8 oz. low-fat yogurt, 2 tbs. low-fat granola
Lunch	400	600	Sliced turkey sandwich, baked chips, banana, nonfat latte
Afternoon Snack	400	300	All-natural high-protein bar or shake
Dinner	400	700	2 small skinless chicken breasts (about 80 grams), 1 cup brown rice, 8 oz. skim milk, 1 cup strawberries, with nonfat whipped cream

Principle No. 3: What to Eat

All six food classification groups are allowed, but you should primarily be eating from Groups 1, 2, and 3. Eat from Groups 4 and 5 occasionally for better overall health, but sticking to the first two principles will usually limit these groups automatically. Your best choices are lean proteins, complex and unprocessed carbohydrates, and either polyunsaturated or monounsaturated fats.

Group 6 falls into the "occasional" and "limited" category. Sometimes you just crave something from this group and nothing can stop you. When this happens, if your overall day still complies with Principles 1 and 2, then there really is no serious damage done. If your daily diet has been compromised by too many bad choices then resume your good habits at your next meal, scale back a bit on your total daily calories the following day, or notch it up a bit at your next exercise session. After all, we are all human. But remember, if you are craving something from Group 6, practice good label scrutiny with processed foods to help keep you on the straight and narrow.

BOK Fat Loss / Weight Maintenance Meal Plan Guidelines for the Six Fuel Groups			
Unlimited	**Occasional**	**Limited**	**Avoid**
Fuel Group / (Acceptable at all meals)	(1 to 3 meals per day)	(1 to 3 meals per week)	(No foods from these groups)
Group 1 — All non-processed foods	All processed foods	—	—
Group 2 — All non-processed foods	All processed foods	—	—
Group 3 — All non-processed foods	All processed foods	—	—
Group 4 — —	All non-processed foods	All processed foods	—
Group 5 — —	All non-processed foods	All processed foods	—
Group 6 — —	All non-processed foods	All processed foods	—

BOK Accelerated Fat Loss Meal Plan

Principle No. 1: How Much to Eat

The first step to accelerated weight loss is eating fewer calories per day. Your daily calories for the BOK Accelerated Fat Loss Meal Plan will be 20 percent less than the BOK Fat Loss / Weight Maintenance Meal Plan. For example, if you need 2,000 calories to maintain your goal weight, you would subtract 400 calories (20 percent of 2,000 calories) to get to your Accelerated Fat Loss daily target: 1,600 calories. Note that this is not a starvation diet. And you will still feel satisfied because you will eat six times a day. Your fuel percentages and ratios are as follows:

BOK ACCELERATED FAT LOSS FUEL PERCENTAGES

(Carbohydrate to protein ratio* is 1:1)

Food size percentages in grams:
45% carbohydrates, 45% protein, 10% fat

Food energy percentages in calories:
40% carbohydrates, 40% protein, 20% fat

*Remember that you can consume the same amount of carbs as protein for both grams and calories.

Principle No. 2: How Often to Eat

As explained above, you will get the best results by dividing your calories equally throughout the day, but only a small minority of people can do this and still remain satisfied. Most people need to vary their calories, though the distribution for this plan differs slightly from the BOK Weight Maintenance / Fat Loss Meal Plan. Instead of five meals a day, there are six, with the addition of a late snack (or part of your dinner saved for this later snack). Lunch should have a caloric value close to dinner and the late snack combined. The late snack should be eaten no less than two hours before bedtime. Also, the calories of the largest meal should be no more than three times the amount of the smallest meal.

Meal	Even Calories	Suggested Calories	Food Examples (for suggested calories
Breakfast	250	150	3 eggs whites, wheat toast with jam
Morning Snack	270	200	Protein bar or shake
Lunch	270	500	Tuna salad (1 can in water) with low-fat dressing, 1 cup black beans, 8 oz. nonfat milk, 1 peach
Afternoon Snack	270	250	8 oz. 1% cottage cheese, 8 low-fat wheat crackers
Dinner/Late Snack	270/270	250/250	Split the following between dinner and late snack: 1 cup whole wheat pasta with 6 oz. lean ground turkey and marinara sauce, 1 cup broccoli, ½ cup fruit salad

SAMPLE BOK ACCELERATED FAT LOSS DAILY MENU (BASED ON 1,600 CALORIES A DAY)

Principle No. 3: What to Eat

The rule of thumb for this plan is to stay within Groups 1, 2, and 3 (unprocessed items only, if possible). The closer you stick to this, the more progress you will make because incidental fat will be introduced into your diet. Complete abstinence of Groups 4, 5, and 6 may not be realistic for you, so try to lean towards foods that contain the healthier fats (monounsaturated or polyunsaturated) and enjoy your other favorites occasionally as long as you keep your fat totals around the recommended 10 percent. To get faster, more consistent results though, try to steer clear of the Fat Cocktails in Group 6.

Also, try to stay away from foods in Group 3 that are simple sugars and select more unprocessed items that offer complex and fiber-rich carbs. Packaged foods will present the biggest challenge so carefully read ingredient lists on labels for hidden sugars, other high glycemic carbs, and salt.

Check out the web site to learn more about planning your meals.

BOK Accelerated Fat Loss Meal Plan Guidelines for the BOK Six Fuel Groups				
Fuel Group	**Unlimited** (Acceptable at all meals)	**Occasional** (1 to 3 meals per day)	**Limited** (1 to 3 meals per week)	**Avoid** (No food from these groups)
Group 1	All non-processed foods	All Processed foods (focus on low sodium items)	—	—
Group 2	All non-processed foods	All Processed foods (focus on low sodium items)	—	—
Group 3	All non-processed foods	All Processed foods (focus on low sodium items)	—	—
Group 4	—	All non-processed foods (focus on low sodium and low fat items)	All Processed foods (focus on low sodium and low fat items)	—
Group 5	—	All non-processed foods (focus on low sodium and low fat items)	All Processed foods (focus on low sodium and low fat items)	—
Group 6	—	All non-processed foods (focus on low sodium and low fat items)	All Processed foods (focus on low sodium and low fat items)	—

LIVING PROOF

Remember our four healthy food groups—fruits, vegetables, meat, and nuts? Well back in the early days of BOK research, the only test subject I had at my disposal was me. And for six months I ate only unprocessed foods from these specific food groups. It was very difficult at first, but my physical health and body composition changed dramatically. I was sleeping better, staying alert longer and my body was much leaner. Even more impressive was how much my laboratory values changed. Bad cholesterol (LDLs) levels plummeted and my good cholesterol (HDLs) increased significantly. Many of my patients have experienced the same results and their doctors agree—food can be good medicine if taken correctly.

BOK Ten Essential Tips for Weight Management

Keeping within your personal total caloric intake, planning five-to-seven meals a day, and eating quality fuels are all keys to making either of these meal plans work. You already have all of the information and tools for you own plan, but here are my top ten tips to help you on your journey. Visit the web site and print this for you and your family to review later or to share it with someone else that might need a little help.

1. Eat when you start to feel hungry.

Note the word hungry. It implies a physiological signal to eat. It has nothing to do with watching television, traditional mealtimes, or feeling bored. As you know by now, once your blood sugar rises and falls, you will physically begin to feel hungry—note the word physically. So, respond. If your machine is working the way it is intended to, you will feel a need to eat about every two or three hours. We are designed to stay on the edge of hunger, eating when our bodies tell us that we need food. We are not designed to eat every meal until we feel full. The new "target feeling" you should be shooting for after a meal is simply the absence of hunger.

2. Drink water before and after meals.

Drinking water at every meal will reduce your calorie intake and bring you to that "absence of hunger" feeling much quicker. Also, water is absorbed more quickly than food, so you won't get that stuffed un-comfortable feeling after eating. Drink water after your meals, too. Remember that your hunger may be thirst in disguise. How much water should you drink? There are two easy ways to find out: Divide your weight (in pounds) in half and that's how many ounces per day you should drink, on average, or make sure that your urine is always on the clear side and not too dark yellow.

3. Make sure you snack at least twice a day.

If you want results that last, snack twice a day. Like any important meeting or errand, set a timer, put it in your day planner, set a reoc-curring reminder on Microsoft Outlook or recruit someone for sup-port until snacking becomes second nature. The choice is simple. You can either try to fool Mother Nature by taking diet pills or skipping meals or work with her by eating five to seven times a day.

4. Minimize your salt intake.

Salt + sugar + any simple carbohydrate adds up to the infamous Fat Cocktail. This fat-friendly combination will result in a higher insulin response and more potential fat storage from each meal. Danger zones are processed foods and when eating out. Read your food labels and choose restaurant items without salt, cream sauces, butter, syrups, etc. Before long you will be fully satisfied with low- and no-salt foods. Re-member salt also makes you thirsty, which can stimulate your appetite. It's no accident that bars serve free salted peanuts, chips, and pretzels.

5. Select complex carbohydrates as frequently as possible.

Whenever possible choose complex carbohydrates and avoid simple carbs—especially in combination with fats. Simple carbs rush into the bloodstream causing a large release of insulin. Higher levels of insulin pack on the pounds faster and will temporarily shut down the body's capability to burn fat as fuel. Choosing complex carbs is a much smarter choice because they usually contain fiber which slows their entry into the bloodstream, which can also prevent some of the fat in your meal from being absorbed and lower the release of the stor-age hormone insulin.

101

6. Eat more carbohydrates early in the day and fewer later in the day.

Try to eat most of your carbs during your first three to four meals on the BOK Fat Loss / Weight Maintenance Meal Plan or your first two to three meals on the BOK Accelerated Fat Loss Meal Plan. An old rule for body builders when "leaning up" before competitions is to stop eating carbs after 3:00 p.m. This will maximize fat burning and minimize fat storage as you sleep. If you must, indulge in sugary carbohydrates only during the daytime when you are active. They are not only burned easier, but the unburned, stored carbs will be available in the evening hours if you exercise.

7. At mealtime, eat some of your carbohydrates before your protein and fat.

If you are feeling famished, your blood sugar is low and begging to be elevated, so give it what it wants first. Start your meal by selecting a small portion of the available carbohydrates (vegetables, fruit, rice, pasta, etc.), wait a few minutes, and then move on to the protein. It takes time for the satiety center in the brain to get the signal that you have eaten (about twenty minutes). And since our brains primarily burn carbohydrates for fuel, this area is more sensitive to carbs than any fat or protein. Even if it takes you only five minutes to eat that small portion of carbs on your plate, it will reach your brain about ten to fifteen minutes later and still slow your attack on the rest of the meal.

8. Eat slowly, chew your food completely, and take short breaks.

Remember the uncomfortable feeling after holiday meals? Not only were your "eyes bigger than your stomach," but your mouth was faster than your twenty minute satiety response time. A simple technique to avoid overeating is to pause at certain points in your meal. Spark up a conversation, or if you are alone, read the paper, check your e-mail, or make a quick phone call. A two to five minute pause a few times during your meal can be the difference between eating normal portions and overeating. Just as important is to chew slowly and completely before swallowing. This too will extend your mealtime and will also help you avoid problems such as indigestion and acid reflux.

9. Make healthy food available.

Take the time to make healthy food available sure that you have healthy snack items available at home, in the car, at school, and at work. Fruit is the best and easiest choice because most come in their own natural wrapping and are fortified with vitamins and minerals. Protein sources are more of a challenge. A few low-fat, high-quality protein fuels that travel easily include whey or soy protein shakes, hard boiled eggs, canned or packaged tuna in water, fat-free / low-fat cottage cheese or yogurt. Of course, meal replacement bars and other prepared items are an easier choice, but remember that they are processed so check their labels first to make sure that you make the best choice. You should always try to make the "natural" choice first, and cooking at home is the most efficient way to monitor your food intake. You control the ingredients and the leftovers are great for lunch or snacks the next day.

10. Reward yourself once a week.

We are all human and sometimes we just want to celebrate life or enjoy other foods outside of our normal everyday healthy diet. Pizza and beer during football season or a good movie with your favorite ice cream may be hard to give up. So reward yourself once a week with something you particularly enjoy, but don't use it as an excuse to "pig out." Keep your more decadent rewards in the 300 to 500 calorie range if possible. Then get back on the program at your very next meal. A little extra exercise can help correct a part of a caloric imbalance, but don't use exercise as a down payment for your next indulgence. Your new healthy you will become your greatest indulgence.

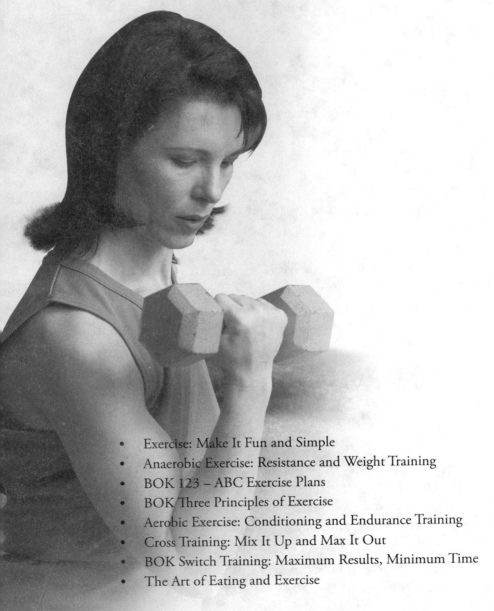

PART 3

ACTIVITY AND EXERCISE

Exercise: Make It Fun and Simple

Pilates, step aerobics, and yoga. Stair climbing, spinning, and running. Circuit, core, cross training, and free weights. There's no doubt about it, physical fitness and exercise have come a long way since kids used to do jumping jacks in the school yard like World War II army recruits. Training techniques today are as diverse as the fitness goals of every individual. From Jack La Lanne to Arnold Schwarzenegger, Jessie Owens to Carl Lewis, Jane Fonda to Denise Austin—the techniques these pioneers helped develop have changed the way we perceive exercise. We exercise not only to feel better but also for fun. The science of exercise physiology offers so many options that it's now possible to get physically fit and be entertained at the same time! Attaining fitness is now easy and accessible. From national chain fitness centers to home gyms, fitness vacations to community walks, fitness has become big business. Getting exercise is now something most people actually love to do.

If what I am saying sounds like a foreign language, there is only one reason: you haven't found the program that's right for you. The incredible array of fitness programs that we have to choose from does have its drawbacks. Some programs are better than others, but most are quite successful in helping you attain the results they tout. If you've tried and failed, don't be hard on yourself. You may have chosen a program that didn't work for your goals and lifestyle. So how do you know whom to believe and where to begin searching for a new program?

First, believe in yourself. Then, begin with the Body of Knowledge guidelines in this section of the book and the corresponding information and programs on the BOKsystems web site. This is the first step to developing the body you want. I can promise you this: you can get in shape, no matter how out of shape or overweight you are right now, and in a way that's comfortable for you. Start by learning about the various exercise options suggested in this section and the effects they will have on your body. Find what you like and what makes sense to you, be honest about your abilities and needs, and set realistic goals. You will be well on your way to building your personal exercise program.

A Fresh Start

The decision of where to start is always the most difficult, especially if you have had your share of disappointments. That's why the first and best place to start is with your mind. Your initial exercise selections should be based on the path of least resistance. The "no pain, no gain" adage does not apply here. If you make informed decisions—and I will do my best to help you—your fitness program will fit naturally in your lifestyle, along with your new eating habits. In addition to all the physical benefits, exercise will help you maintain a certain level of mental clarity and peace of mind. If your exercise program becomes a source of stress, that is the first clue that you need to reevaluate the program you've selected.

The second step starts in front of your bathroom mirror. Look at yourself and really think about the physical results you want from an exercise program. You must be realistic. You can influence your shape through certain exercises, but they will not produce results overnight or give you a body just like someone else's. What results, you must ask yourself, are realistically attainable for you? Consider other factors. Are there any physical barriers that might limit your abilities? Any health problems? And don't forget to consider your age. Trying to keep pace with twenty or thirty-year-olds when you are sixty-something may not be attainable, safe, or healthy.

Notice that I did not say anything about getting on a scale. That's because I want you to forget about it. You will lose weight as you lose fat, but you'll also gain and tone muscle, which, pound-for-pound, weighs more than fat. In this sense, the scale can work against you if your lean and fat mass ratios change to healthier levels. So, use the scale to track your progress in the beginning stages, but eventually replace it with your senses of sight and feel. How do you look? How are you're clothes fitting? They are not only better indicators of your success and progress, but you'll be able to manage your results without being stressed by numbers on a scale.

> WHAT RESULTS ... ARE REALISTICALLY ATTAINABLE FOR YOU?

Now, back to the mirror. Mentally strip away the flesh and picture what's naturally underneath. Your basic structure or morphology is the one thing you cannot change. Though we all vary due to our genes, science recognizes three general body types, called morphological shapes: endomorph, ectomorph, and mesomorph. They are so named by the dominant body tissue type (ectoderm, mesoderm, and endoderm) inherent during early fetal development.

Mesomorph   Endomorph   Ectomorph

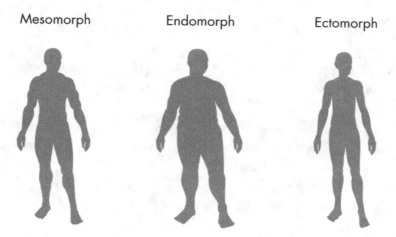

Telling an endomorph that it's a piece of cake to look like a supermodel ectomorph sets unrealistic expectations and is a setup for ultimate failure. However, with the knowledge you gain from the BOKsystem, you can modify your basic morphology. Though you can't change your basic skeletal structure, you can change the shape of the tissues that surround it.

> When you hear about body shapes, do any celebrities immediately come to mind? They did for us, check out the web site to see who fits the profiles and why.

So, why am I telling you this? Because being realistic and honest with yourself will be a key to your success. I want to encourage you to be the best *you* can be. I don't want you to give up before you begin because you believe that your DNA is working against you. It isn't— or at least it doesn't have to. I too have tried and failed at exercise, but I was fortunate enough to discover why and learn how to develop a program suited to my needs and goals. My goal is to assist you in your own search to find the program that will work best for you, and make it a positive experience.

Aerobic Versus Anaerobic: Fueling Around

Aerobics became a household word in 1968 when Dallas researcher Kenneth H. Cooper, MD, coined the term, which resulted from his research showing that heart-pumping exercises, such as running, can condition the heart and improve cardiovascular health. It set off a fitness revolution that has not abated. Before aerobics became a noun, the adjective aerobic was simply a scientific term used to describe the metabolic activity within the muscles that is required to support physical conditioning and endurance. Translated, aerobic metabolism means "activity requiring oxygen."

The opposite of aerobic is anaerobic, and it describes the metabolism needed to support strength and speed. Translated, anaerobic metabolism means "activity not requiring oxygen." Though the word anaerobic never became a household word, it is just as important as aerobic when it comes to true fitness.

As you learned in Part 1, metabolism is the mechanism by which energy (ATP) that we get from food is produced. Hence, the well-known phrase metabolic rate means the speed at which energy is created and fuel is burned. And that brings us back to the core theme of this book: helping you understand the importance of energy—where it comes from, how you use it, maintain it, and burn it—to reach your health and fitness goals.

Energy—Again?

That's right. We are back to energy because, so far, I've only told you half of the story. As you learned in Parts 1 and 2, all body cells depend on carbohydrates, protein, and fat as fuel sources. They make up what scientists call potential energy. These fuels, however, do not have the ability to come out of storage and go into action on their own. Their potential energy must be converted by our metabolism to that energy-carrying structure—ATP.

> **QUICK DEFINITIONS:**
>
> **Aerobic** means "with oxygen"
> **Anaerobic** means "without oxygen"

When we work our muscles through exercise, the demand for energy increases—they burn and call for a larger supply of ATP. In essence, the energy equation I explained earlier (to make ATP from carbs and fats) is accelerated during and after exercise. And since ATP is used up quite rapidly, it needs to be replenished continuously, which burns more of the fuels stored in and around your body.

The Metabolism–Exercise Connection

Let's take a look at the key players in energy production and clear up some of these terms. Food supplies aerobic and anaerobic metabolism to make the energy, ATP carries the energy, then your aerobic and anaerobic exercise burns the energy.

It's that simple, but how and why do you switch between aerobic and anaerobic? There is only one substance that determines whether we use more aerobic ATP or anaerobic ATP: *oxygen*. With oxygen we are able to burn fuels in our aerobic metabolic machinery to make ATP; without oxygen, we get ATP mostly from our anaerobic metabolic machinery. Think about how much oxygen a marathon runner uses in comparison to someone who breathes less working out with weights for a shorter amount of time.

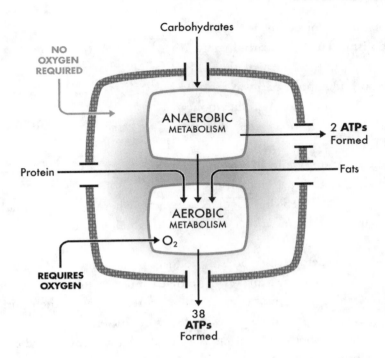

At any given time both metabolisms are running to produce ATP. Steady breathing and low-intensity exercise keep oxygen flowing on its aerobic metabolic pathway. But if you quicken your step or hold your breath during some strenuous exercise, the oxygen supply to your cells will diminish and anaerobic metabolism kicks in.

Why, you must be wondering, is this so important? Because aerobic metabolism runs primarily on fat and anaerobic metabolism uses only carbohydrates. This gets us to the real reason behind this scientific excursion. If you want to burn fat, you need to work aerobically. But if you want to improve your ability to burn fat faster and keep it off easier, you have to work anaerobically, which involves burning some carbohydrates in order to build metabolism-boosting muscle.

Burning Fat and Carbs

Although there is plenty of research describing the positive effects of aerobic activity on the heart, another benefit is that exercising aerobically burns more fat. Conversely, anaerobic activity utilizes carbohydrates to help build that fat-burning muscle. While pro-

teins are involved in aerobic metabolism, fats and carbohydrates
directly produce most of the ATP
for both metabolic pathways. Both
anaerobic and aerobic metabolic
pathways make the same quality
ATP, but the quantity differs significantly. If you would like to know
more, check out Metabolism In

> AEROBIC METABOLISM
> RUNS PRIMARILY ON
> FAT AND ANAEROBIC
> METABOLISM USES ONLY
> CARBOHYDRATES.

Motion on the web site [icon] to see exactly where the ATP is made,
how it is made, how much is made, and which area of metabolism
is making it.

Because aerobic metabolism produces much more ATP than anaerobic metabolism, it makes sense that it must utilize a heavy-duty
battery charger like fat, which supplies more than twice the calories
per gram than protein or carbs. In terms of efficiency, it then makes
sense that the body chooses fat as a fuel during long, sustained exercise. Unfortunately, that means when it comes to burning excess fat, it
requires a longer time commitment from you.

The good news in all of this is that we don't have to work harder
or more intensely to burn fat. That's because if you work your body
too hard—that is, if you work it to the point where your breathing
becomes difficult—your metabolism will switch to anaerobic metabolism, and you'll flip from burning fat to burning carbs. It seems that
with such "sensitive" metabolisms, we would be able to switch from
burning one fuel to another quite easily in order to burn all of the
fat that we want, or all of the calories. We can—but it isn't as easy as
flipping a switch. There's more to it. It's important to remember that
although aerobic metabolism favors fat fuel, it burns some carbohydrate fuel too.

My point? Both aerobic and anaerobic metabolisms burn carbohydrates. And unlike fat, carbohydrate stores are in limited supply.
If carbohydrates are depleted, everything shuts down, including our
ability to burn fat. It is called "hitting the wall," a condition of exhaus-
tion that you sometimes see in athletes attempting superhuman feats
like marathons and triathlons (I cover this in greater detail later in this
section).

It is possible to purposefully and effectively decrease the stores of a certain fuel by maintaining an aerobic or anaerobic metabolism, but you need to attain a physical balance you can "feel" in order to make this happen. It takes time and a certain level of conditioning, but once you reach that point, you will be able to burn more fat, ingest different combinations of fuels to help maximize your workout, and improve your overall diet, exercise, and weight management outcomes.

Let's review what each type of training has to offer individually, as well as in combination, to help you create your exercise plan.

You have two kinds of muscle: fast and slow "twitch." Find out which twitch helps you burn fat and which helps you burn carbs on the web site .

Anaerobic Exercise: Resistance and Weight Training

If your goal is to shape and tone your body or improve your metabolism, then you need to incorporate some type of anaerobic exercise into your life. The physical expression of anaerobic exercise is resistance training, or working out with weights. It is the kind of exercise that tones, builds, and strengthens muscles.

There are many benefits to having toned, well-developed muscles. Taut muscles are incredibly efficient at metabolizing calories. That's because more muscle mass means more metabolic machinery. More machinery naturally burns more fuel, even when at rest. It's a perk you don't want to miss out on.

Resistance training will also help your endurance training. Studies have shown that stronger muscles obtained through anaerobic exercise increase the staying power required for aerobic activity. With added weight training, endurance exercises will feel easier to perform and your aerobic staying power will receive a boost. Resistance training also promotes joint stability, increases tendon strength, and makes bones stronger—all-important to your overall health as you age. Rather than letting your muscles atrophy and bones soften, you can literally defy aging by putting up a little resistance.

Forget the old stereotype of some hulking mass hoisting a 300-pound barbell over their head while grunting. He Tarzan? Maybe. But it certainly isn't you—and it definitely is not what you typically

see in gyms today. Today's gyms are
filled with average Joes and Janes
of all ages and shapes going from
weight machine to weight machine
or free weight to free weight solely
to attain the benefits of resistance
training.

> RESISTANCE TRAINING
> WILL ALSO HELP YOUR
> ENDURANCE TRAINING.

Going to the "max" is not what it is all about anymore. People
often tell me that they become frustrated by weight lifting because
it is too hard and it takes too long to feel the results. I unfortunately
have to agree with them, because if it is too hard and you are not getting results, it means that you are not doing it right. You are wasting
your time.

BOK Three Principles of Exercise™

The irony of weight training is that it is not all about the weight.
Rather, in order to yield better, faster, and more lasting results—no
matter what type of resistance or aerobic training you select—you
must understand and master three very important basic principles:
repetitions, technique, and breathing. This is what weight training
and all resistance exercise is really about.

WEIGHT RESISTANCE FOSTERS AGE RESISTANCE

Working your muscles yields enormous benefits as you age. Physical abilities are both enhanced and limited by the strength and flexibility of our muscles. Ignore your muscles by not using them and they will atrophy, along with the joints, ligaments, and tendons that work together to protect your muscles and provide a natural range of motion. The deterioration in your ability to perform physically will be subtle during your twenties, thirties, and possibly even into your forties, but you'll begin to notice monumental differences as you enter your fifties and beyond. Joint and muscle aches and pains will set in, and gradually the degenerative joint disease known as osteoarthritis can develop. Bones can also lose their strength and become brittle, leading to the debilitating disease known as osteoporosis.

Sounds depressing, doesn't it? Well, these so-called diseases of aging do not have to happen. Studies show that older people who perform weight-training exercise on a regular basis combined with a healthy diet have the same bone or muscle mass as people twenty years younger or more. In one study, researchers found that just one to two days a week of resistance training increased muscle mass and neuromuscular performance for women sixty-five to eighty years of age. Other studies have shown similar findings for men. Another important benefit for older men and women is the potential for reducing the risk of falls or fractures.

Principle No. 1: Repetitions

How much ya benchin', dude?
Hey, buddy, what's your max?

Translated, this gym lingo means, "How much weight can you lift at one time?" In technical terms, it refers to the maximum weight that one can displace on an apparatus such as the bench press. It's the quintessential Tarzan image that we mentioned and associate with weight lifting. For some unknown reason, the bench press has become the icon for weight-lifting superiority (mainly with us guys), promoting the false idea that more weight is better. If you are training for a sport that requires excessive strength and speed in a particular muscle group, then your max is relevant. Otherwise, max should not be your concern.

There is an old rule in weight lifting that still bears truth: using lighter weights will give muscles more tone, and using heavy weights will increase muscle size and strength. At the end of the day, though, the number of repetitions is more important than the amount of weight. For better, lasting results, I want you to focus on repetitions—the number of times you can lift the weight.

A repetition is the ability to complete one full motion in which a particular muscle group is contracted or shortened and then relaxed or elongated. The average number of

> THE NUMBER OF REPETITIONS IS MORE IMPORTANT THAN THE AMOUNT OF WEIGHT.

repetitions, or "reps" for any particular maneuver is about ten to fifteen without having to rest. If you can't or can barely do that many repetitions without straining intensely, then you might be using too much weight. You should use the amount of weight that enables you to perform the specified repetitions, with the last two to three repetitions requiring some extra effort. With that said, you don't want to make it too easy either.

So, how do you know when you are ready to ratchet your weight up a few pounds? It's purely a judgment call. After a few weeks at the same weight, add some more. If the last two or three reps greet you with a little resistance, then you've hit it right; if they are a big struggle, drop down to a more manageable amount of weight. Think of it as sugar in your coffee. Add too much all at once and you'll ruin the whole cup; add just a little at a time, tasting as you go, and you'll hit your perfect balance.

Principle No. 2: Technique

Technique is the most influential factor when it comes to the quality of muscle development and maintaining your results. Proper technique ensures contraction and elongation of a particular muscle group by putting it through its proper range of motion and doing it correctly. I cannot emphasize the word correctly strongly enough.

Bad technique can result in asymmetry, meaning a muscle group may develop out of balance compared to the same group on the opposite side of your body. Your arms for example, could each develop a different size, shape, and strength. Bad technique can also mean that it will take you more time to get the results you want. More commonly, poor technique means not reaching your goals at all, which could cause you to become discouraged and

> PROPER TECHNIQUE IS THE MOST IMPORTANT FACTOR WHEN IT COMES TO MAINTAINING RESULTS.

quit. Worst of all, bad technique can result in injury that could set you back for weeks, months, or longer.

Good technique is not difficult to achieve. It begins with a certain level of simple coordination before you can give it your all. The important thing is to avoid developing bad habits at first, because they will be hard to break later.

I could tell you how to do your reps correctly, but if you find someone, either a personal trainer or other certified expert, to give you hands-on instructions a few times, you will minimize mistakes. You can also consider taking a class. Many gyms today offer classes that focus on resistance training, and the instructors will guide you through the exercises. There are specialty centers for women, seniors, and children too. You will be far more successful if you learn how to do it right before you start out on your own.

Contraction Dynamics

Mention the following two technical terms to a trainer and they will be duly impressed. Contracting your muscles is one half of what technique is all about. You will actually be putting your muscles through two different contractions: concentric and eccentric. For you acronym lovers, they are known as the CC (concentric contraction) and the EC (eccentric contraction).

The CC is the exercise emphasis, or main effort that tightens and shortens the muscle against resistance. The best-known example is the classic pose of flexing the muscle in the upper arm, the bicep. Think Popeye after downing a can of spinach. Conversely, the EC is the returning effort that releases and elongates the muscle against resistance (usually gravity combined with the weight) through a controlled return to the starting position. It's a harder type of muscle contraction to understand than the CC, but an excellent example without using weights is the simple walking stride. When the heel of the foot strikes the ground in front of the body, the lower leg muscle group in front (the group situated to the outside of your shin) releases those muscles with an EC contraction to place the foot on the ground in a controlled fashion. Without an EC, your foot would slap down uncontrollably on the ground with every step.

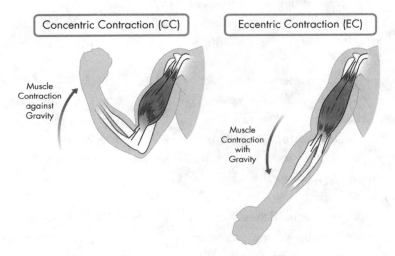

Range of Motion

Range of motion—ROM in exercise nomenclature—is the second half of the technique equation. It is a term you are probably already familiar with because it is inherent in so many aspects of everyday life, such as getting in and out of a car, or other activities that you perform without thinking about them. With weight training, however, you must pay particularly close attention to your ROM.

During any particular exercise, it is important to maintain a healthy range of motion that is neither too short nor too exaggerated. For example, there is more to ROM of the biceps muscle than the traditional flexing Popeye pose. You must find a complete but comfortable range of motion which brings the forearm in contact with or as close as possible to the upper arm (CC). And then on the return, you must continue the motion in a controlled fashion (EC) until the arm is almost straightened out. Although contraction dynamics is important for results, it is also important for safety. With an improper ROM, not only are you setting yourself up for pain later on, you are risking a muscle tear, ligament strain, or other injury. The idea is to find the ideal median between the average ROM and your unique, healthy ROM.

The musculoskeletal system has limitations on its end ROM. (It's the extraordinary, rather than the ordinary, who can perform those incredible yoga twists.) Bones, joints, and ligaments are all involved in ROM. Every individual is different, so you need to become familiar with your personal ROM and how far you can take it. Avoid extremes but experiment with caution until you find your own healthy range of motion.

Even at the microscopic level, ROM is important—in fact it makes more sense. You know we need ATP to fuel both contraction _and_ relaxation, but did you know where? Our individual muscle fibers are not single, continuous units like nerves or other structures. They are made up of many tiny units called _sarcomeres_ that contract and relax together to control your ROM. Go to the web site to see how they work.

Proper technique also includes the entire body. While you are exercising any group of muscles, there are other muscles performing important contractions that do not involve movement; this is called stabilization. The stabilizing position of your feet and arms, the way you hold your back and head, and the speed at which you do your repetitions are just as important as the way you execute targeted muscle movement. These factors are all part of technique and need to be included in your learning process. Good technique also requires an elevated level of focus. Mastering technique requires effort, but it is what produces the best results.

Principle No. 3: Breathing

Don't hold your breath!

When you start lifting weights, make this your mantra: breath in, breath out. People tend to hold their breath when doing something strenuous, although they are often not consciously aware of it. It's common, and as you learned earlier, our anaerobic metabolism will only provide us with a limited supply of ATP in these breathless (low oxygen) situations. If you are concentrating on your proper range of motion or pushing a little harder on your last few repetitions, you may hold your breath without realizing it. To avoid this, try to focus your attention on your breathing, not the weight, until it becomes an integral part of the very motion you are performing.

Your breathing should not be exaggerated, but kept steady and full. The best technique is to inhale through your nose as you release and lengthen the muscles you are working (EC) and then exhale through your mouth when you tighten and shorten (CC) them. Believe it or not, this breathing helps the heart and lungs actually "pump" more oxygen to your muscles and waste products (like carbon dioxide) out of your lungs. Check out the web site to see an illustration that shows you how correct breathing makes all of this work. Do not force your breathing too hard in either direction. Avoid short breaths (panting) or holding your breath, even for a few seconds. Suspended breathing suspends oxygen. As mentioned previously, oxygen is important because it dictates the type of metabolism your muscles select, which in turn dictates the kind of fuel you burn and limits the amount of energy (ATP) available for exercise.

BREATHE AWAY BURNING AND SORENESS

Since your ability to resistance train is driven by anaerobic metabolism and limited by carbohydrate fuel supplies, stopping your breath will only boost the need for more carbs and use them up faster. With carbs in short supply in your body, this could mean a crash in your energy level and a premature end to your workout. It also contributes to the buildup of lactic acid, a metabolic waste product of anaerobic activity. Lactic acid (see the section "Burning and Fatigue" in Part 5) is what causes muscles to burn during your workout and can contribute to greater soreness following your workout. And if you are holding your breath because of pain or difficulty, you are better off trying a different exercise or lowering the amount of weight you are using.

Choose Your Weapon

So, how do you start?

Start slowly. This is always my answer when it comes to any new activity or specific exercise. It is the prudent approach that produces the best—and most lasting—results.

What should you start with first?

Now we're getting into an area of some debate. Every personal trainer or exercise enthusiast is asked, "Which is better—free weights or exercise machinery?" "Health club or home?" A good answer should be, "A little of both, but whatever works for you."

The truth is, when starting out, the type of weight training and location will not affect your final outcome very much. Either free weights or machines, at the gym or at home will help you achieve noticeable muscle tone, the goal of most beginners.

Most weight machines are great for resistance training, but they don't always produce the same results as working out with free weights. The easiest way to explain this is with the natural way gravity and muscle function together. The body develops naturally as a result of its response to gravity, so it makes sense that more natural movements that make use of gravitational forces are best suited to maximize your exercise results. This should always give free weights the advantage, but some machines are designed to closely mimic these natural movements and are very effective. Your choice depends on your own individual goals and expectations.

Free weights (more specifically dumbbells and barbells) are a smart choice if you are interested in increasing your tone, coordination, muscle mass, and improving shape. It's a "better bang for your buck" situation because they are as reliable as the gravity that governs them. They are also the most versatile because they can be used at home or in a gym. And a set of light dumbbells can even go with you when you travel. Their biggest drawback is safety. An initial training program is usually necessary to understand and maintain proper technique. While most weight machines keep you locked into a strict range of motion, your knowledge and coordination are the only things governing your ROM when you use free weights. Ignoring proper technique can result in poor outcomes or injury.

Free weights are so effective because in order to perform exercises that concentrate on particular muscle groups, you depend upon the strength and stability of other muscle groups to support them. For example, strong shoulders are necessary for an efficient chest, back, or arm workout. This muscle group is the main stabilizer of the connection between the arm and the torso. And a strong, stable torso (chest, back, abdominals) is crucial for an efficient extremity workout (arms and legs). Strong, developed arms conversely provide the grip and stability necessary for an efficient upper torso workout (chest, back, and shoulders).

> FREE WEIGHTS ... ARE A SMART CHOICE IF YOU ARE INTERESTED IN INCREASING YOUR TONE, COORDINATION, MUSCLE MASS, AND IMPROVING SHAPE.

This multi-muscle connection is the reason working out with free weights tends to be more difficult than working with weight machines, especially in the beginning. But this phenomenon happens in other types of exercises as well. Walking, running, biking, push-ups, and pull-ups all use more than one muscle group. The addition of weight increases the resistance for all of the groups involved with that particular exercise, instead of isolating a single group, as some machines do.

Today there is a whole line of machines that mimic gravity and maximize muscle contraction. These machines are better than some of the older models at increasing the stress on particular muscle groups and helping to increase size, shape, and strength. Some even have different positioning capabilities. If you commit to using a weight machine, get proper instruction and make sure it is available when and where you need it to maintain consistency in your workouts.

Although I may seem to favor free weights for increasing muscle size and improving shape, you should do whatever works best for you. Both weight machines and free weights build and shape muscle mass quite efficiently, and mixing the two is a good alternative if they are both accessible. Give either choice a chance though; only trial and error will deliver true answers and tangible results.

Timing Is Everything

No matter what you use to exercise, you need to use it regularly but not too frequently. Your muscles are designed to respond to a certain amount of effort and then recuperate for a particular amount of time. Giving your muscles time to rest between certain exercise sets and workout days is crucial to success.

REST FOR SUCCESS

Because weight training is an anaerobic activity and primarily burns carbohydrates for fuel, it is difficult to continuously push through set after set without tiring. The rule of thumb for working the same muscle group is to rest thirty seconds to two minutes between sets. This will give the worked muscle group time to recover and replenish its supply of ATP for the next round. Pushing a muscle group to the point of fatigue is another way to maximize size and strength, but pushing past fatigue to complete muscle failure early in your development will increase the risk of injury. When toning, the time between individual sets is not as crucial and can be as short or as long as you desire. If you use the BOK Switch Training™ technique (described later in this section), rest time will automatically occur when you move on to another group of muscles.

In the same way that resting between sets helps hold off fatigue and reenergizes your muscles for better performance on the next exercise, resting muscle groups three to four days between workouts is critical to your overall results.

The physical act of an exercise is only part of what is required to achieve the size, strength, and mass you desire. The actual building process takes place after the workout, when the muscle is at rest. It is the three phases of injury, recovery, and repair that are necessary for the growth and development of a muscle. Weight training strains your muscles and creates minute tears in muscle fibers. Three to four days of rest for individual muscle groups allows time for the normal recovery and repair phases. The repair process results in a firmer, stronger muscle.

GIVING YOUR MUSCLES TIME TO REST BETWEEN...WORKOUT DAYS IS THE KEY TO SUCCESS.

And muscle will always try to grow stronger to prepare for an effort that is similar or greater than the one previously required.

How long should you wait between workouts? The answer is: do not focus on your entire workout program, but the individual muscle groups involved in each training session. Wait three to four days between workouts of individual muscle groups. For example, if you work on your chest and back muscles one day, you could work on your legs or arms the next day, or even the same day. But whatever combination you choose, make sure that the groups you work have time to respond and repair before you work them again.

A simple way to discover your individual repair-and-development period is to wait until a specific muscle group is no longer sore before exercising it again. If you wait too long, though, the muscle group will begin the process of atrophy, meaning its mass and strength will begin to decrease.

If muscle toning is your goal, muscle atrophy is not a factor since muscle firmness and maintenance are the goals. In fact, if you only work each muscle group once a week, the two to three days of exercise neglect will not be noticeable or even felt with a good toning program. As I said previously, getting the results you want may not require as much of a time commitment as you thought!

Whatever your goal, do not underestimate the power of rest. It's a lose-lose situation if you don't rest and a win-win if you do. Read on to learn about this issue in Part 5; "Muscle Plateaus—What to Do When You're Stuck." I'll show muscle building enthusiasts a better way to use rest and muscle memory to surpass these stubborn levels of muscle strength or development.

So now that you know the basics, it's time to get down to the specifics. Weight training can produce a variety of different results and there are many ways to achieve them. The information you'll find in this book will help you make decisions about the different types and frequencies of exercise by explaining how and

> THE THREE PHASES OF INJURY, RECOVERY, AND REPAIR ... ARE NECESSARY FOR THE GROWTH AND DEVELOPMENT OF A MUSCLE.

why different approaches work. I will also recommend a few types of exercises and exercise schedules. Pick one that suits you the best or use one as a foundation that you can modify to create your own unique program.

The key to success is to find something that works for you and your lifestyle. Only you know what you want and need. Understanding how to achieve the results you want will help you adapt an exercise plan to your goals and needs.

MUSCLE MEMORY

Muscles grow and adapt to prepare for future efforts similar or greater to what they've been put through before. Because of that, once you reach a certain level of muscle development and strength, your body will be able to return to that same level if you become too busy to work out for a few days, weeks, or months. Your muscles will actually remember their previous level of development and have the ability to return to the same level of development faster and easier than the first time you worked to achieve that level. This *muscle memory* will stay with you for the rest of your life once you have resistance trained and maintained a higher level of muscle development.

BOK 123 – ABC Exercise Plans

Before we get into exercise specifics and your preferences, I would like to introduce you to a weekly exercise planning system that incorporates all of the information you have learned up to now into nine easy plans to choose from. The BOK 123 – ABC classification will allow you to pick a level of comfort, match it to your present schedule, and also give you the ability to adapt to future goals. The numbered plans correspond to the total days per week you choose to exercise and the lettered plans give you the option within those total days to choose how many days you would like to resistance train. You can select from a list of many different conditioning (aerobic) exercises and resistance (anaerobic) training exercises, but I recommend that you incorporate the BOK Switch Training technique we will discuss later into your plan.

The plans follow a simple numbering system that involves a minimum and maximum daily exercise requirement for the week:

Plan 1 – Exercise four times per week
Plan 2 – Exercise five times per week
Plan 3 – Exercise six times per week

Each plan has options A, B, and C that correspond to the amount of resistance or BOK Switch Training performed during the week. And by default, the amount of conditioning days are the remaining days per week left over from the total days exercised in the plan number chosen:

Option A – BOK Switch Training two times per week
Option B – BOK Switch Training three times per week
Option C – BOK Switch Training four times per week

The following is an example of BOK Exercise Plan 1-A. Go to the web site to see all nine of the plans and sample exercises.

BOK Exercise Plan 1-A

- 2 days per week Switch Training
- 2 days per week short Aerobic exercise
- 2 days per week long Aerobic exercise
- 3 days of rest

Day	Type of Exercise	Weight	Sets	Repetition/ Duration
Monday	Total Body Switch Training Short Aerobic Exercise	Light —	1 —	10–12 reps 15–20 minutes
Tuesday	Rest			
Wednesday	Long Aerobic Exercise			20–30 minutes
Thursday	Total Body Switch Training Short Aerobic Exercise	Light —	1 —	10–12 reps 15–20 minutes
Friday	Rest			
Saturday	Long Aerobic Exercise			20–30 minutes
Sunday	Rest			

Making Muscle

No matter where you are on the fitness scale, your muscles can be primed for toning, building, and, if you really get into it, sculpting. Toning is not about big muscles; it's about firm muscles. And you can achieve firmer muscles, as well as other perks—such as flexibility, endurance, and structural integrity—through easy, enjoyable exercises that require just a few hours a week. Muscle building on the other hand, is all about muscle size or lean mass. It requires dedication and time initially, but the more knowledge you gather, the sooner your workouts will feel like a good habit that you have been enjoying for years.

Both muscle toning and building can be achieved by using the three principles of exercise (appropriate repetitions, correct technique, and proper breathing) discussed in the last section. But both still require an initial level of coordination and a certain level of commitment to understand how to achieve results. There is a sharp distinction between learning, experiencing, and knowing. A little trial and error will help bridge the gap between the first two, and the latter is directly connected to your results. Once you learn how to develop your muscles, the next step is to experience the outcome. This is what the initial education or coordination phase of resistance training is all about—your muscles' ability to respond to the exact commands sent by the brain. It is important to begin gradually. Go back to the beginning of this part of the book if necessary, and reread the information on technique, repetitions, and breathing. Focus on truly knowing the importance of these elements of effective exercise and the results they produce. Jot down a few notes about your likes and dislikes in your BOK Journal or in the margins of the BOK 123 – ABC Exercise Plans™ that you have printed from the web site. This information will be valuable during the initial phases.

Remember to keep your mind on your breathing and vary repetitions and weight according to your goals. Sometimes it is better to start with one to two sets of an exercise using an amount of weight that does not challenge your muscles too much. Just going through the motions for the first few weeks could put you ahead of those who work too hard trying to make up for lost time.

Make sure you warm up your muscles first with some stretching or five to ten minutes of walking, slow jogging, biking, or other low-level aerobic exercise. If this is your first time weight-training, enlist the help of a personal trainer or another knowledgeable person to help you select exercises that will work both your upper and lower muscle groups. Or you can refer to the web site ▭ for more information about specific exercises. If you do have the resources, a trainer can show you the correct way to use machines and/or free weights. It is wise to follow up with them in a month or two to see if you have forgotten anything or started to develop dangerous habits. You must gain the proper knowledge to yield better, faster, and lasting results.

Augment your resistance program by taking a class in yoga, stretching at home, or participating in some other physical activity centered on a healthy range of motion and breathing techniques. This is an important step that will help you minimize soreness, avoid injury, and feel a sense of accomplishment during the initial stages of a new exercise regimen. Also, select initial resistance exercises similar to the ones you want to perform later. After you improve your coordination and stamina, you can safely and comfortably move on to a greater amount of weight and other more challenging exercises.

Muscle Toning: Start Your Engines

This is where personal preference begins with your BOK exercise plan. Although exercise and eating habits are both important and necessary for weight management and better health, you have a choice on which you would like to focus more time and effort. Firming and toning your muscles is really all anyone needs to do, since most of your health and fitness results weigh heavily upon healthy eating habits. Working on toning your muscles can be a lot of fun, it doesn't take a lot of time, and you will enjoy the results because you will actually be able to see and feel the difference right away!

If you have never done any type of resistance training, weight machines are a great place to start. A trainer might also suggest some exercises using light barbells, and many gyms offer body sculpting classes that also focus on toning exercises. Be sure to choose classes that are designed for beginners or all experience levels. The important thing is to develop a program that works all of the muscle groups one to two times a week, which will be sufficient in the beginning. Start slowly by doing one set of ten to fifteen repetitions for each exercise with light weights. Keep in mind, once again, that technique is critical. Add your own exercises one at a time and spread them around the week in an effective, comfortable manner. Otherwise, you can use the one of the sample BOK 123 – ABC Exercise Plans that give you the option of four to six days per week of total exercise with a mix of two to four days per week of resistance training as a starting point. If you choose to try your own plan or one of the examples without out professional training, be sure to continuously scrutinize your technique. Focus on your movements and the three principles of exercise, and watch yourself in the mirror to check your form. Your emphasis should be on avoiding bad habits and injuries at this stage.

> FIRMING AND TONING YOUR MUSCLES IS REALLY ALL ANYONE NEEDS TO DO.

In just a few weeks, you will begin to notice a difference in your muscle tone, coordination, and strength. Don't, however, allow that progress to give you a false sense of security. Structures such as tendons, ligaments, and joints take longer to adapt to a new activity. Try to resist a premature acceleration into heavier weights or more sets and repetitions. Concentrate on stretching and maintain your beginner's program for at least six to eight weeks.

Toning requires only a level of resistance that produces mild fatigue at the end of each set of repetitions. And your muscles should only feel tight and tense a day or two after your workout, not too sore. If they do feel very sore, you are working too hard, and you could be undermining your results. An exception to this is for those who have never attempted any type of resistance training or were sedentary for an extended amount of time. After your first few sessions, the initial soreness will subside quickly.

If indeed tone is all you desire, just enjoy your workout at a relaxed pace. After your initial six to eight weeks you can increase the number of sets, but try not to do more than three sets per muscle group, more is simply not necessary for a toning program. You can begin to vary the amount of weight as well. You can also vary the number of repetitions depending on the muscles being exercised, but try not to exceed thirty or drop below ten reps per set. This goes back to the "better bang for your buck" theory. For example, your triceps and shoulders would probably get the same toning effect from vacuuming your living room as you would from performing more than thirty repetitions with very light weight. The only muscle group that will benefit from more than fifty repetitions are the abdominals (your stomach muscles).

THE ABOMINABLE ABDOMINALS

Of all the muscles in the body, the abdominal muscles or "abs" seem like the hardest to develop, and for two good reasons. They do not increase in size or change shape as much as other muscle groups and they do not become easily visible until the layer of subcutaneous fat around your midsection is reduced. The BOK web site will show you how a combination of proper technique, the right number of repetitions, and even correct breathing can quickly firm up and develop your abdominals and help you get rid of that spare tire around your stomach.

As you approach your goal, it will become easier to maintain your muscle tone or push it up a notch by adding a little burn—enough to feel it during your last two to three repetitions. Keep in mind, however, that soreness a couple of days later is not necessary for a maintenance level exercise program. You should shoot for the feeling of firm, tight muscles. As long as you maintain a consistent workout regimen, the effort you expend need only be minimal—even once or twice a week can keep you where you want to be. Once your toning plan becomes routine, you can experiment with dietary changes and concentrate on time efficiency. And when you reach this level of comfort, there is an unexpected benefit I call "unconscious compliance." If you are enjoying both the effort and the results, you will continue your workouts without extensive planning or sacrifice.

Sample Muscle Toning Weekly Schedule

The following is a beginner's muscle toning plan that mixes anaerobic with aerobic activity on alternate days with added abdominal exercises. During your resistance or BOK Switch Training days, you should use light weights and do only one set per muscle group one to two times a week for the first six to eight weeks. Then, as your muscle coordination, education, and confidence improve, you can begin to gradually increase your weight and number of sets. After a few months, you can follow the three to four day workout rule between muscle groups, and your weights should be heavy enough that you feel mild to medium resistance during your last two to five repetitions.

BOK EXERCISE PLAN 1-C:

- 4 days per week Switch Training with short Aerobic exercise
- 4 days per week short Aerobic exercise
- 3 days of rest

Day	Type of Exercise	Weight	Sets	Repetition/ Duration
Monday	Upper body Switch Training	Light	1	10–12 reps
	Abdominals	—	1	15–50 reps
	Short Aerobic Exercise	—	—	15–20 minutes
Tuesday	Lower body Switch Training	Light	1	10–12 reps
	Abdominals	—	1	15–50 reps
	Short Aerobic Exercise	—	—	15–20 minutes
Wednesday	*Rest			
Thursday	Upper body Switch Training	Light	1	10–12 reps
	Abdominals	—	1	15–50 reps
	Short Aerobic Exercise	—	—	15–20 minutes
Friday	Lower body Switch Training	Light	1	10–12 reps
	Abdominals	—	1	15–50 reps
	Short Aerobic Exercise	—	—	15–20 minutes
Saturday	*Rest			
Sunday	**Rest			

* These days can incorporate either aerobic exercise or rest, according to your weekly schedule and goals.

** Suggest additional abdominal work out here to maintain the effective two days on and one day off cycle.

Another time-effective variation of this routine is to do both upper and lower body exercises on the same day, two to three days a week. This plan, like the others, is versatile. For beginners you can leave the plan as is and then gradually substitute twenty to thirty minutes of light aerobic activity for one or two of the rest days such as walking, slow jogging, biking, or skating—anything you enjoy enough to continue on a regular schedule.

Muscle Building: More Mass Burns More Calories

Although there are many new options available these days for all types of exercise, the old rules of muscle development still provide better, more consistent results. The size of muscle you build is directly proportional to the amount of weight used and the number of repetitions completed. It's that simple. If you want to increase your muscle mass, you must increase the amount of weight you are using. But as you increase the weight, you should decrease the number of repetitions and intensify your focus. It shouldn't be a harder workout, just different. Initially, it will seem like you are doing more work, but when the size and strength of your muscles catch up, it may feel easier, quicker, or more satisfying than any toning workout. But remember, if you are a beginner, you need to start with a toning program before working on a more advanced muscle-building program. Give your bones, tendons, and joints two to three months to adjust before substantially increasing the weight you use in this type of muscle building program.

Muscles are not primarily built by increasing the number of fibers (or cells) within each muscle. Rather we increase the size of our muscles by increasing the size of individual muscle fibers. And to do this you must incorporate the proper combination of technique, repetitions, breathing, and rest into your lifting program. Otherwise, your results will be mediocre at best. The way your body sees it, the purpose of muscle building is to match the strength of muscle to the load placed upon it. More developed muscles can handle more resistance and more resistance requires more developed muscles.

> MORE DEVELOPED MUSCLES CAN HANDLE MORE RESISTANCE AND MORE RESISTANCE REQUIRES MORE DEVELOPED MUSCLES.

I believe that honesty is the best policy, so again I am letting you know that in the beginning, you *will* feel soreness. In fact, you want to feel a little soreness because it indicates stress on the muscle groups you want to develop. And our bodies have instructions to develop stressed muscles in order to overcome and avoid that same level of stress in the future. Remember, though, that my definition of "sore" is a level above "tightness" and is not associated with the old adage "no pain, no gain." You should be able to move easily and should only notice the soreness when you are using the muscle group you worked previously. Just keep moderation as your workout mantra and use a "spotter" to help you with new techniques.

SEE SPOT HELP

A spotter is someone trained in muscle building techniques and who is present to prevent accidents, injuries, improper technique, or to help you safely push yourself to a higher level. As a beginner, your trainer will be your spotter. If you choose not to use a trainer, find somebody to exercise with who has some experience with spotting who can help you in the beginning. Their job is simple: teach the proper technique and make sure you don't hurt yourself.

Once you have gained a comfortable level of coordination and strength and no longer consider yourself a beginner, you will be able to perform most of your exercises on your own. It is a good idea to check your form and technique with a trusted source from time to time though. Keep in contact with this source for this reason, but progressing to a higher level of strength and size can also require a spotter. If you advance by either increasing your weight or using the same amount of weight and increasing your repetitions, use your spotter to help you complete the last one or two repetitions. "Help" is defined as offering a minimal amount of force that enables you to continue and finish the tightening and shortening contraction (CC).

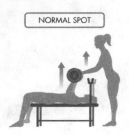

NORMAL SPOT

Other strength training techniques include the "Pyramid" training method and "negatives," which involves a spotter. Check out the web site to see these techniques and others.

Push and Pull

This type of workout I am going to describe for you is one that strength trainers have been using for decades. It is a traditional technique that works the same group of muscles during a single training session.

Because muscle size will respond to a heavier stimulus and to micro-muscular injury caused by the heavier workload, then directly or indirectly working harder will build more mass. But this doesn't mean working out more frequently; remember you must still rest to rebuild muscle. This traditional technique works all similar muscle groups in the same workout.

Most muscles have either a common pushing (extension) or pulling (flexion) function in relationship to the torso.

Main Muscle "Pull" Groups	Main Muscle "Push" Groups
Back (latissumus)	Chest (pectorals)
Front of the arms (biceps)	Shoulders (deltoid)
Front of the hips (ilio-psoas)	Back of the arms (triceps)
Back of the thighs (hamstrings)	Buttocks (gluteal)
Front of the lower legs (extensors)	Front of the thigh (quadriceps)
Stomach (abdominals)	Calves (gastrocnemius-soleus)

The strategy for this technique is to work either push or pull groups during one session or day. You can work all your push or pull groups or just select areas, but one central core group and one extremity group is the minimum requirement. The theory is that it will increase size and strength by continuously stressing all of the muscle fibers within the push or pull group. For example, the pectoral, deltoid (front part), and tricep muscles are all in the push group and are in the upper body. So, you would start with a pectoral exercise, then move on to the deltoids and finish with the triceps, working your way from your core out to your extremities.

Each individual exercise works the muscle on which you are focusing, but it also works the other two because their movements are connected to each other. For example, when you work out your chest on the bench press, the muscles in your shoulders and arms also contract, but are not working as hard as your pectoral muscles. The larger muscles of the torso also share the workload (because they are stabilizing) when you're working your triceps and deltoids individually.

Because all of the muscles in a group are in continuous contracting mode during these types of exercises, they are naturally overworked and you may feel some initial fatigue, especially in the extremities. But in no time, strength will overcome the fatigue. The following is a weekly sample that shows a traditional muscle building and strengthening schedule using this technique. It may not be my favorite anymore, but it does produce results.

My advice is that you don't start your exercise program until you finish reading the rest of parts 3 and 4, then follow up with Part 5 to avoid any of the usual setbacks. And with the aid of the web site you can create and manage your exercises according to your lifestyle and individual needs.

SAMPLE TRADITIONAL MUSCLE BUILDING WEEKLY SCHEDULE

Day	Muscle Group	Weight	Sets	Repetitions/ Durations
Monday	"Push" Groups	Moderate to heavy	3–5	8–10 or pyramid
Tuesday	"Pull" Groups	Moderate to heavy	3–5	8–10 or pyramid
Wednesday	Rest			
Thursday	"Push" Groups	Moderate to heavy	3–5	8–10 or pyramid
Friday	"Pull" Groups	Moderate to heavy	3–5	8–10 or pyramid
Saturday	Rest			
Sunday	Rest			

Muscle Sculpting: Fine Tune Your Efforts

I want you to know that there are other, newer techniques for muscle building that allow you sculpt and shape your body while you become more physically fit. As you gain strength, knowledge, and confidence, you can begin to concentrate on the exercises that you instinctively know will give you the best results in the areas that you want to improve the most. It is the epitome of what BOKsystems is all about—personal empowerment through knowledge of how to create your own program.

After you have been performing a particular routine for a while, you will begin to notice which muscle groups require less attention and which require more. If you continue to learn new exercises, test them out, and change your workouts accordingly, you can vary your performance and shape.

This is called muscle sculpting, a combination of muscle building and toning techniques to help you shape any part of your body you want.

There are ways to get closer to your ideal body. It does take time and attention to detail (more so than what I've described so far), but we will introduce you to the latest exercise techniques that provide you with results faster and with less effort. We will explore these and combine them with eating habits for real life examples in Part Four, where we start Putting It All Together. Tuck this idea away in the back of your brain and return to it when you feel that you are ready to devote more time and energy to your workouts. It's time now to turn your attention to increasing your aerobic capacity and get on a track to better cardiovascular health and burning more fat.

> MUSCLE SCULPTING...
> SHAPE ANY PART OF YOUR
> BODY YOU WANT.

CHANGE IS GOOD

The last tip for muscle building and development is to change your exercises during the week or a few times a month. A muscle's response to stress is a response to a change in activity. Performing different exercises with the same muscle group will constantly challenge your muscles and produce better results. Studies show that muscles will remain at the same size and strength after a certain amount of time if you continue to repeat the same exercises. That's good for those who are happy with their results and want to maintain them, but not for those seeking progress. No need to work out harder and longer; just take a break from your program and try a completely different exercise and watch the way your muscles respond.

Aerobic Exercise: Conditioning and Endurance Training

Oxygen is Mother Nature's most amazing gift. Even though we can not see, feel, or smell this simple gas, it is responsible for our very existence. We inhale it into our lungs, where it is packaged and distributed to our cells. Every vital process sustaining life requires oxidation, which is the processing of oxygen. Whether we are burning firewood for warmth or burning fat in our bodies to make ATP, oxygen is the chemical key. It also plays a vital role in aerobic conditioning and in how our bodies burn calories.

Aerobic metabolism (defined as "with oxygen") is the kind that primarily burns fat. Therefore, a lack of oxygen can impede or completely stop aerobic metabolism. If exercise is too intense, or if you are breathing incorrectly, oxygen will be less available, and the body will abruptly switch to anaerobic metabolism (defined as "without oxygen"), which is the kind that likes to run mainly on carbohydrates. Oxygen is the metabolic key that activates this switch quite easily—a dramatic demonstration of the importance of steady breathing when exercising aerobically. Oxygen availability is crucial in obtaining the twin benefits of aerobic exercise—burning fat and maximizing endurance. Fat is burned in the presence of oxygen and that extra ATP produced is necessary for the endurance that uses it. It also minimizes your fatigue and allows you to better enjoy aerobic exercise.

While I personally love what weight training does for my body and weight management, I enjoy aerobic activity the most. I save some of my favorite aerobic activities for the weekends and other times when I want to relax. I can't think of any type of exercise more enjoyable than going for a peaceful run on a cool, cloudless morning. It is something I treat myself to two to four times a week. A relaxing run, walk, bike ride, or roller blade outing will not only help shed that extra layer of fat around your middle, it will also release natural feel-good endorphins (Mother Nature's mood elevators and pain killers). It will also strengthen your heart, keep your arteries clear, boost your immune system, help you sleep more soundly, increase mental clarity, reduce stress, and even enhance your sex life. It will also keep your fat-burning metabolism revving for hours afterward. Plus, it just makes you feel great for the rest of the day. Exerting energy to earn energy—what a great concept!

To get a handle on what aerobic exercise is all about, we need to start with the heart.

Target Heart Rate

Target heart rate is discussed pretty much anywhere where good health is a topic: at the doctor's office and posted on outdoor bicycle paths and in gyms. Computerized treadmills and stationary bikes are even programmed to calculate it for us. But what does it mean? Our target heart rate lets us know when we are working our hearts too hard or not hard enough and is also an indicator of the main type of fuel we are burning—carbohydrates or fat. Here's how it works:

Even if you maintain deep and steady breathing, the load or effort you place upon your body and cardiovascular system dictates the availability of oxygen. If you push yourself too hard during exercise—above your target rate—you will use up the oxygen available to your muscles too fast (and switch to anaerobic metabolism). The only way you can get more oxygen from the bloodstream is to breathe more efficiently, slow down your exercise intensity, or both. When it comes to dictating the flow of oxygen, the heart and muscles overrule the lungs. "Running out of breath" or "getting a second-wind" are probably familiar terms to you. Go to the web site [📖] to find out how this is connected to your target heart rate.

Maintaining your target heart rate helps keep the heart, lungs, and muscles cooperating for peak oxygen exchange. Your target heart rate is the number of heart beats per minute you must achieve and maintain to sustain oxygen-based aerobic metabolism. As your heart rate increases, the rate at which you burn fat increases until it reaches an optimal point—this is called your threshold rate. If you push the heart too far beyond this optimal point, your body will switch to anaerobic metabolism and call on its carbohy-

> **When it comes to dictating the flow of oxygen, the heart and muscles overrule the lungs.**

drate stores for extra energy. Since carbohydrates are in limited supply (especially if you have been exercising in this manner for more than an hour or did not eat many carbs that day), you will tire and not be able to maintain your aerobic exercise for very long.

The mistake most people make is pushing too hard, believing that if exercising aerobically burns fat then pushing harder will burn more fat. Not so. If you push yourself to the point at which your breathing is labored, you have probably surpassed your "anaerobic threshold" and are no longer burning fat. Exercising at a fat-burning target heart rate requires minimal effort.

What's Your Target Heart Rate?

Your target heart rate is unique, so an absolutely accurate determination necessitates medically conducted testing. But unless you are a world-class athlete, you only need an approximation of your target heart rate to be sure that you are in the right range.

Let the web site [www.] calculate your target heart rate for you.

You will be amazed at what little effort it takes to maintain your target heart rate. A quick and easy test is to see if you can talk while you perform an aerobic exercise at your target heart rate. If you are gasping for breath or even skipping sentences, take it down a notch or two until you can read aloud or finish a conversation. Problems will only arise if you exercise inconsistently throughout the week or push too hard in the initial stages. Remember that pushing too hard is counter-productive. Even worse, it is possible to push yourself to the limit where your body actually runs out of fuel and shuts down and you are physically unable to go any farther. This is rare for most people, but long distance runners (especially marathon runners) know the feeling all too well. It is called "hitting the wall."

HITTING THE WALL

Even if you're a lean, fit machine running at your optimal pace, you are not running on fat alone. Carbohydrates are always contributing to your energy level. In fact, the process of burning fat depends upon a certain amount of carbohydrate consumption to keep you going. Because the body stores carbohydrates (glycogen) on a limited basis, it is necessary to continually supply this fuel. It is the reason athletes "carb load" before a long-distance event. Even at a steady target heart rate, prolonged exercise can deplete carbohydrate stores. For example, when runners run too far or run out of carbohydrates, they "hit the wall" and physically cannot take another step. It means neither aerobic nor anaerobic metabolism is functioning, and that means there isn't enough ATP to contract or relax their muscles. It can be a serious situation that can even lead to a loss of consciousness. So for those of you who like to really "cut out the carbs," you may want to reconsider before you hit the gym or track.

Target Fat Burning

The really cool thing about aerobic exercise—and the big benefit if you're trying to trim down—is the way your target heart rate can help shed fat. As you now know, aerobic exercise turns on aerobic metabolism, utilizing oxygen to burn fat, which provides you with energy. Rise too far above your target heart rate, though, and metabolism can switch to carbohydrate-burning anaerobic metabolism. In fact, the two metabolisms switch back and forth all day long, depending on your activity. Aerobic activity usually has the upper hand because it provides so much more energy (ATP) when it burns fat and remains the dominant metabolism while you are at rest.

Burning fat, however, does not kick in the moment we step on the

> EXERCISING AT A FAT-BURNING TARGET HEART RATE REQUIRES MINIMAL EFFORT.

treadmill or take off down the road. During the first five to ten minutes of aerobic exercise, you will predominantly burn carbohydrates. So, if fat loss is one of your main concerns, you must exercise beyond ten minutes—twenty to thirty minutes is good, and forty-five to sixty minutes is the best, once you are in good physical shape. (The Institute of Medicine recommends sixty minutes of physical activity per day.)

What I find most impressive is that aerobic metabolism will continue to burn fat after you exercise, even if you are just sitting at your desk at work. It's like getting paid double time without working overtime! After an aerobic workout, your metabolism can remain elevated for up to twenty-four hours. As for scheduling and timing, you can do your aerobic exercise anytime during the day, but doing it before your biggest meal or two hours after are the best choices. If you exercise around lunch, you can enjoy the fact that your exercise is done for the day and you will still burn more calories throughout the afternoon.

Walk "In" Your Dinner

A good walk after dinner is another great way to help fight fat. It burns calories, but more importantly it will help prevent fat production and storage. As you know, eating releases insulin (the storage hormone) into your system. The bigger the meal, the more insulin is released, which is likely to turn any extra protein, carbohydrate, or fat from your meal into stored fat. Go for a relaxing walk after a meal, however, and you can do much more than turn on that fat-burning metabolism. The stroll around the neighborhood turns on a chemical reaction that pulls carbs out of your bloodstream and converts them into glycogen, which is stored carbs to be used as energy at another time. And with fewer of those carbs around after your meal, there is less insulin released. This is good for two reasons: First, you'll have more stored carbohydrates for mental and physical activities later. Second, the carbs from your meal going to glycogen storage won't be going to contribute to fat conversion or storage. Grab your wife, husband, partner, friend, kids, or organize a neighborhood walk after dinner and watch your waistline shrink!

Let's Get Started

Even if you have been in great aerobic shape in the past, there is nothing to be gained by starting out too fast or too slow. An exuberant beginning may initially burn more calories, but it isn't worth the potential for injury. So be patient. Don't try to make up for lost time! If you were in shape before, your performance will accelerate faster (remember muscle memory) than if it's your first stab at aerobic activity. And if it is your first attempt at aerobic conditioning, you'll be surprised at how quickly you will progress.

Take time to choose the best exercise for you. Choose something that you enjoy and that fits your lifestyle, so you'll be more inclined to do it on a routine basis. As your heart, lungs, and musculoskeletal system adjust to your new activity, you can advance to a higher level. Loving what you are doing and feeling and seeing the results will take the "work" out of your workout.

If you are out of shape, have never tried aerobic exercise before, or have been away from this type of exercise for several months or more, follow this advice: Take two steps forward and one step back. Just like resistance training, advance slowly and make sure you rest a day or two when you feel soreness, stiffness, cramping, or the unusual fatigue that may be associated with your new activities. Your body will let you know if you are overdoing it. Listen to your body! If you adopt this attitude you will reach your goals comfortably and be far more likely to maintain them.

> YOUR BODY WILL LET YOU KNOW IF YOU ARE OVERDOING IT. LISTEN TO YOUR BODY!

How often should you work out aerobically?

Answer: Three or four times a week is ideal, but no less than twice and no more than six times a week. Make sure you start off at a comfortable level of exercise. If aches and pains are bothering you, skip a day or even two if necessary. If you feel fatigued rather than invigorated afterward, take it as a sign that you are doing too much at once or need a different schedule throughout the week.

You must be able to maintain your target heart rate without extreme soreness, fatigue, or loss of breath before you increase the amount of time you exercise and the intensity of your workout. You should start out slowly so you can maximize your carbohydrate stores, which will maintain your target heart rate for a longer period of time. Once your body becomes accustomed to a longer time period, your heart rate will eventually decrease as your body becomes acclimated and your conditioning improves. To return to your optimal target rate, you can either quicken your pace or increase your effort.

If you are returning to aerobic exercise after a prolonged absence or injury, follow the Rule of Thirds: Begin your exercise regimen at one third of your usual distance, time, and intensity for at least one week. Add another third only after you have had an entire week without pain or unusual discomfort. If you do experience any ill effects or symptoms of overexertion, simply scale back to your previous weekly training level or rest until they have passed. Once you are at a comfortable level again, you can advance your intensity and time duration another third until you have reached your original level or new goal.

Here are a few suggestions for weekly aerobic exercise:

Every Other Day

If intensity is not your style, this is a great schedule. It is also great for beginners who can benefit from a day of rest between workouts. It will minimize the chance of injury and allow for variation in future intensity. For example, if you are feeling a little stiff or sore from a previous strenuous session, you can do a light day or easy session two days later. By the next session, you should be ready to resume where you left off four days earlier. Four days between more intense sessions is plenty of time for tissue regeneration and repair.

Once you find your level of comfort, the every-other-day cycle creates a work and reward experience. For every day of effort there is a day of regeneration, offering a comfortable, restful feeling.

5 Days On, 2 Days Off

This is the most popular regimen because it parallels a regular work week. Aerobic exercise is one of the best stress relievers around, which is why most health clubs are crowded at lunch and after work. Many

146

people like to keep their work and exercise schedules in the same cycle so that their weekends or days off can be totally carefree.

Like the every-other-day option, you can alternate long and short or fast and slow days. I suggest that you also vary the type of exercise performed throughout the week. This is another way to rest certain structures and muscles while continuing to exercise. For example, biking the day after a long walk or run will rest and reduce the impact to your hips, knees, ankles, and feet, but will still provide an excellent aerobic workout.

One Long, One Short, One Rest Day

This schedule has the greatest potential to produce the best results with the fewest problems. It is popular with serious fitness buffs, as well as those who work their aerobic exercise in with an existing anaerobic, resistance-training regimen (cross-training). Your can also maximize your abdominal (stomach) exercises on this schedule. One high-effort day followed by a low-effort day and one day of rest is an ideal way to give muscles a better opportunity to repair and strengthen.

Cross-training: Mix It Up and Max it Out

Wouldn't it be nice to gain muscle mass, lose fat, have more endurance, decrease your time in the gym and get better results than people who are slaves to a conventional workout? If you think so, you are not alone: you are part of a growing majority that has adopted an exercise technique called cross-training. Cross-training is an exercise platform that combines anaerobic and aerobic exercise. As you now know, resistance (anaerobic) and endurance (aerobic) training can be used to achieve different physical results and fitness goals.

Anaerobic exercise promotes strength and speed; aerobic exercise promotes cardiovascular conditioning and endurance. Cross-training simply combines the two in a strategic plan that allows you to exercise more efficiently. You can perform your conditioning before weight training or weight train first and then condition, or alternate the two (for example, change every fifteen minutes during a one-hour workout). There is really no right and wrong way to cross-train; just find the method that gives you the results you want and in a way that you enjoy. Another big benefit of cross-training is that it can easily accommodate your lifestyle. It allows you to customize a results-oriented program to suit your schedule and appeal to your personal interests. It offers something for everyone.

Cross-training can take the highly-motivated exerciser to a higher level and it can turn an exercise-phobe into an achiever. The only rule is that it must include a combination of resistance training and aerobic conditioning exercises. There are endless exercise routines that you can create, which will give you variety, to keep you interested and engaged. Through cross-training, you can better prepare yourself for obstacles that may stop you from exercising. If you have any aversion to aerobic workouts in crowded classrooms or other routines that make your lungs burn, your heart pound, and your muscles ache, take heart—there are endless choices for activities that provide aerobic exercise.

Take on a recreational activity, such as skating, tennis, or walking, after your weight-training session. Aerobic exercise does not have to be difficult or unpleasant. Hate the thought of going to a gym? Then purchase a few hand weights and plan an anaerobic program you can do at home, or take them to another location where you can incorporate the aerobic activity you enjoy into a cross-training session. These suggestions will put you on a sensible and effective track to fitness and will produce results quicker than older, more conventional exercise plans.

> ### WHICH COMES FIRST: CONDITIONING OR WEIGHT LIFTING? FIND OUT ON THE WEB SITE.

So, you can see how versatile cross-training can be. You can make it work for you whether you are too big, too small, too fat, too skinny, too busy, too tired, too shy…the list goes on and on. Personally, I love cross-training because it offers everyone a chance to get the results they want and maintain them. It's a way to stay fit in less time and within the demands of your unique lifestyle.

A specific technique I have developed, called BOK Switch Training, offers all of the benefits of cross-training and more.

BOK Switch Training: Maximum Results, Minimum Time

BOK Switch Training is the epitome of smart exercise. It works muscle groups just as well as any conventional workout program but does it in a way that saves time and offers better overall results.

As you know, conventional weight-training programs focus on specific movements that target one or two muscle groups during a single training session. This method requires that you physically stop all activity and rest between sets while your muscle endurance and strength recover. BOK Switch Training, however, allows you to perform the same muscle stimulating exercises, but without requiring the downtime or rest between sets—and without making you feel like you need one. Instead of stopping all activity between sets or exercises for a particular muscle group, you switch back and forth between opposing muscle groups. This inherently saves time since you are removing all the resting; recovery times between sets during your workout session. It probably shaved twenty to thirty minutes off of my workout the first time I tried it. BOK Switch Training involves the push and pull muscle groups we discussed earlier, but we added a research-based technique that involves switching back in forth between opposing muscle groups called *agonists* and *antagonists*.

OPPOSITES ATTRACT

When performing arm curls, the biceps are the agonist muscle group and the triceps are the antagonist muscle group. Then, when the triceps are exercised, then they will become the agonist and the biceps become the antagonist. Check out the web site [icon] for exercise examples of different body parts where you can combine these techniques to create your own plan.

Agonist–antagonist BOK Switch Training allows you to continue exercising without stopping because the antagonist muscle group is naturally at rest while its agonist is at work. Studies show that working muscles in this way can actually offer strength-building benefits similar to longer conventional resistance training programs, while also enhancing endurance. Furthermore, the muscle will have a larger range of motion and it will be easier to stretch before and after exercise. Special nerve receptors in our muscles and tendons shut down the antagonist while we are working the agonist. All of our muscles have this natural reflex that keeps them relaxed so they (antagonist) do not fight against the agonists' contraction. BOK Switch Training requires that you alternate using the following muscle group examples. I recommend that you start with the push muscles when possible.

PUSH		PULL
Chest (pectoral)	↔	Upper back (latissimus)
Front shoulders (anterior deltoids)	↔	Rear shoulders (posterior deltoids)
Back arms (triceps)	↔	Front arms (biceps)
Lower back (Erector Spinae)	↔	Stomach (abdominals)
Buttock (gluteals)	↔	Hip flexors (iliopsoas)
Rear thighs (hamstrings)	↔	Front thighs (quadriceps)
Calves (gastrocnemius-soleus)	↔	Front leg (extensors)

BOK Switch Training takes advantage of another phenomenon passed down to us from our ancestors. Any of your antagonist muscles will have a more forceful contraction and fuller range of motion right after their agonist counterparts have finished their contraction. It turns out to be a survival trait going back to primitive times. For example, when we are running from danger, there is a trading off of contractions between our opposing leg muscle groups—the quadriceps and hamstrings. (Those who didn't most likely became dinner for a saber-toothed tiger.) The same holds true for our upper body. If there is an obstacle in our way, like a ledge or fence, we must pull ourselves up with the pulling muscles (latissimus and biceps), and then push ourselves over with pushing muscles (pectorals and triceps). Bottom line: BOK Switch Training naturally creates an all around better and more natural workout.

BOK Switch Training also introduces a conditioning element to your resistance training. Although working an agonist muscle group allows the antagonist group to recover or rest, the continuous switching effort causes an increased load on the heart and lungs. Switching from one group to its opposite without rest allows you to sustain an elevated heart and breathing rate, thus providing an aerobic component to your anaerobic weight-training session. So BOK Switch Training will not only get you out of the gym faster, but will also help you burn fat!

Another beautiful thing about BOK Switch Training is its versatility. Even if you are in a crowded gym with someone using the next weight station in your exercise plan, you can simply skip ahead to another body part. I try to maximize my efficiency and minimize resting (and socializing) by planning my path at the gym and making sure that the weights and machines are available. But if you just finished working your chest and someone is occupying your favorite latissimus pull-down machine, substitute another back exercise or move on to your legs and do a back-to-back set with your quadriceps and hamstrings. You can always return to your back and chest later. I assure you that your heart will not slow down a bit!

> BOK SWITCH TRAINING WILL NOT ONLY GET YOU OUT OF THE GYM FASTER, BUT WILL ALSO HELP YOU BURN MORE FAT!

You can do an abbreviated aerobic workout after BOK Switch Training, too, and save a longer aerobic program for the days you do no resistance training at all. However you divvy it up, this type of training will save you time and help you produce noticeable results.

It is also the ideal program for weight management and fitness maintenance.

There are two main ways to apply the switch-training workout. One is an intensive approach, where you get maximum results over a short amount of time. Believe me, it's a program that delivers but is only for the seriously dedicated. But maybe you're like me (usually pressed for time) and need a less intensive or more time-efficient routine. I find that the older I get, the less time I have to spare. These days, my free time is a fraction of what I had when I was younger. At first, my workouts suffered. Then desperation became the mother of invention, and making the most of the time I had became my new goal. All I wanted was to maintain my fitness level while spending less time in the gym and on the track. So I came up with a few time-efficient routines that were also result-efficient. One time-efficient plan requires two long days, three short days and two days off. The long days include a heavy resistance program that works out all of the major muscle groups, followed by a light aerobic workout. The short days are for long runs or rest with more attention to my eating habits. The long days take dedication, but what the heck, it's only twice a week!

To see more details about this plan, how to get around obstacles, and also check out a more intensive weekly schedule, log on to the web site.

The following is just one sample of a time-efficient weekly schedule:

BOK EXERCISE PLAN 2-A

- 2 days per week Switch Training
- 2 days per week short Aerobic exercise
- 3 days per week long Aerobic exercise
- 2 days of rest

Day	Exercise	Weight	Sets	Repetitions/ Duration
Monday	Total body Switch Training Short aerobic exercise	Moderate —	2–3 —	8–15 reps 15–20 minutes
Tuesday	*Long aerobic exercise			30–45 minutes
Wednesday	*Long aerobic exercise			30–45 minutes
Thursday	Total body Switch Training Short aerobic exercise	Moderate —	2–3 —	8–15 reps 15–20 minutes
Friday	*Rest			
Saturday	*Long aerobic exercise			30–45 minutes
Sunday	*Rest			

*Any combination of aerobics and rest is possible depending upon time constraints and individual priorities.

Before You Begin, Warm Up and Stretch

Don't start out with cold muscles and stiff joints! To really reap the benefits of your exercise routines, it is very important to warm up first and stretch your muscles. Warming up and stretching your muscles, tendons, joints, and ligaments is essential because it decreases your chance of injury and discomfort after exercise. The elastic and inelastic qualities of muscle tissue can withstand only a certain amount of stress, and if they are not adequately prepared, damage can result. Preventing injury, however, is not the only reason you need to warm up and stretch. It will also improve your comfort level during exercise. You may feel subtle differences in your flexibility and range of motion in your twenties, thirties, and forties, but the differences and limitations can be monumental in your fifties, sixties, seventies, and eighties. While others are humped over, shuffling around, and complaining of stiffness, aches, and pains, you will have more spring in your step and more fluidity in your movements.

Notice that I say warm up and stretch. They are two different processes with a common goal. Warm up your muscles with at least five to ten minutes of gentle aerobic exercise of any kind, even walking is just fine. The objective is to increase your blood circulation and heat things up a bit to make your muscles and other supporting structures more pliable.

CROSS-LINKING: A CHEMICAL REACTION OF AGING

Stretching is essential to maintain the elasticity of body tissue as you age. Elasticity offers shock absorption, much like the shocks in a car. Even more important is its ability to assist in storing "potential energy." Like a rubber band, when fibers are stretched during activities, they absorb and store energy (potential energy) that can be used when they spring back to their original length. The only thing that influences this is the aging process.

There is a chemical process constantly at work called *cross-linking*. This process causes the fibers or structures that would normally stretch or slide past each other to bind together (via a molecular bridge) This cross-linking bridge limits normal movement, and with time the fibers can bind together into a stiff structure that has next to no elastic capabilities. Your only defense against cross-linking is to break them before they form—and that means consistent warm-ups, cool-downs, and stretching with exercise.

Stretching is altogether different. The amount of time you spend stretching is up to you, but proper technique and timing are as vital as performing the stretch itself. A proper stretch involves a "static" or constant force applied to the muscle group. Don't bounce or push your stretch once you have reached the end of your range of motion. Stretch to the point where you feel the tension or slight discomfort in your muscles and tendons, hold it for ten to twenty seconds, and then release. Repeat the process two or three times per muscle group.

Your range of motion will improve with time but here's an additional timing technique that will improve your stretching, right from the start. The most effective way to stretch is to first flex, or consciously contract (CC) the muscles or group to be stretched then relax them. The short recovery stage after a contraction relaxes your muscles briefly and allows them to stretch more, creating a greater range of motion during your stretch. The final stage of this stretching technique is to contract the opposite muscle group while you are holding your stretch. For example, the body automatically relaxes the hamstring muscles more if you contract your quadriceps (upper thigh). Lastly, don't forget to breathe throughout the stretch. Holding your breath will not help you and may restrict your stretch by allowing metabolites to accumulate. The proper stretching sequence overview is as follows:

> PROPER TECHNIQUE AND TIMING ARE AS VITAL AS PERFORMING THE STRETCH ITSELF.

Contract muscle group (agonist) → Relax muscle group (agonist) →
Stretch and hold → Breathe and contract opposite muscle group (antagonist)

Perform each stretching cycle three times before and after exercise. If you only have time to stretch before or after, stick to the one that gives you the best results. The web site has a demonstration of a proper calf stretch using this technique.

The Art of Eating and Exercise

One of the most commonly asked questions I hear is, "What do I eat when I exercise?" A better question is what and when you should eat in regard to exercise.

The individual food items and food combinations you eat will vary depending on when you exercise and what kind of exercise you choose. Again, as with most things in this book, there are no hard and fast rules. There are a few practical guidelines that you should follow though to make smarter eating and exercise choices.

Eating Before Exercise

If fat loss is your primary concern, eat very little before aerobic exercise. After the first five to ten minutes of activity at your target heart rate, your body will pull primarily from your fat reserves. Before breakfast is a popular time for conditioning exercises, but two to three hours after your most recent meal will work just fine, too. The only time you may want to eat a little more before aerobic exercise is if your body's stored carbs (glycogen) are already low as a result of earlier aerobic exercise or after heavy anaerobic resistance training. You'll know this is happening if you feel the signs of low blood sugar, such as fatigue, agitation, or light-headedness. A simple carbohydrate or complex carbohydrate with a small amount of protein, such as fruit and oatmeal or a low-fat dairy product, can give you a quick boost and will not hang around in your stomach as long as other heavier foods.

Eating before resistance training is easier to explain—just do it! Remember, this exercise depends on a short supply of carbohydrate fuel. It also preys upon the very muscles (amino acids) you are trying to build and maintain. You can't beat a soy or whey protein shake with fruit before you hit the weights, but a turkey, lean beef, or tuna sandwich will do just as well. Just make sure you eat an hour or two before you start training to avoid cramping or reflux (heartburn).

Eating During Exercise

Some people work out harder and/or longer than others. If you are planning to do an hour or more of aerobic or anaerobic exercise, your body will continue to perform better if you give it some carbs after this duration. Try the vast selection of sports drinks while you are working out. These products have come a long way from their sugar and water forefathers. Most have some electrolytes (sodium and potassium) and a few varieties now contain some protein or amino acids. Just experiment with the different mixtures, see how you feel during your workout, look for any changes in your results, and find what works best for you.

Eating After Exercise

As for eating when you are finished with your exercise, one study found that a 3:1 carbohydrate-to-protein ratio is optimal for muscle repair and growth. Eating immediately after exercise is more important when doing resistance training, but you also need to refuel after aerobic conditioning. If your emphasis is on muscle development, you can eat simple carbohydrates to get your best insulin response. I eat a simple and/or complex carbohydrate along with protein in a 2:1 weight-maintenance ratio to ensure that my muscles always have enough goodies to repair, build, and maintain their mass while minimizing my caloric intake.

I recommend that you eat after you exercise no matter where you are in your daily calorie intake. It is more important to give your body and muscles what they need since you can always slack off on calories at the next meal or next day if your focus is fat loss.

Combine one, two, or all three of these eating and exercise suggestions until you find the perfect blend of exercise, food, fun, and results. I use both before and after suggestions when I weight train by eating a quick 2:1 or 3:1 carb-to-protein snack one to two hours before I work out and then a smaller snack with the same ratio within fifteen to thirty minutes of finishing.

LOW-CARB ISN'T ALWAYS THE ANSWER

If your goal is to step your exercise regimen up to a higher performance plane, you should not be on a very low-carb diet. Some people can do it, but if the lower carb and exercise combination is not comfortable for you, then I do not recommend it. Any increase in activity will burn more carbohydrates. Although you may have plenty of fat to supply your aerobic exercise routine, remember that your carbohydrate reserves are always limited. You don't want to run out and end up "hitting the wall," the potentially hazardous condition I described in the chapter "Aerobic Exercise."

The 60 percent carbohydrate ratio (gram weight) that is part of the BOK Weight Maintenance/Fat Loss Meal Plan will keep your physical and mental efforts running smoothly if you weight train a little harder or condition for longer periods of time. If you are exercising harder, but your focus is still on maximum fat loss, the only thing you should reduce is your fat calorie intake and then slowly reduce your total calorie intake as tolerated.

If you feel confident with the information you have been given in this section, try a few variations to see what works for you, because it's time to make your own plan. But if you would like to begin with something tried and true first, simply choose one of the eating and exercise programs in the next section, Putting It All Together, as your foundation. Tailor it to your personal needs and preferences as you experiment with diet and exercise plans. Continue to modify it according to your goals and results. In the end, it will be your plan.

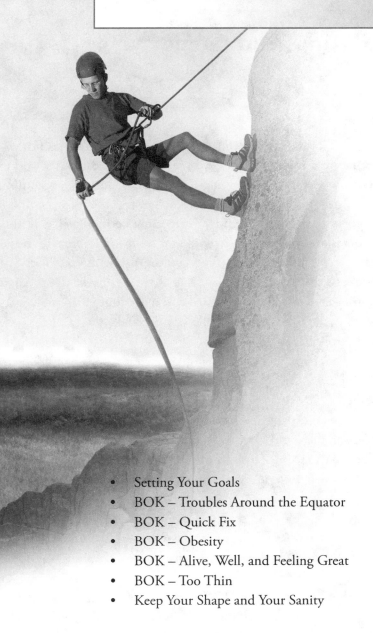

PART 4

PUTTING IT ALL TOGETHER

Setting Your Goals

Now that you have an enhanced knowledge of diet and fitness—facts and fiction—I hope you feel empowered to start working on your own Body of Knowledge health program. As you continue reading, select the eating habits and exercise suggestions that work the best for you. The BOKsystem is so appealing because it is so flexible. Some of you may design a program and stick with it forever; or you may add and subtract certain food choices or exercise methods until you are satisfied with the results. That is the beauty of the program. You can take what you have learned and meet your goals while working within your lifestyle. It also allows you to adapt your plan as your life and goals change.

First, let's explore the ease of implementing a personalized dietary plan using the BOK Three Principles of Eating as a foundation. The guidelines in Principle No. 1 for how much to eat are easy to follow, and you can adjust your caloric intake until you find the right number to fit your short-term and long-term goals. Obviously, that number will change from time-to-time, but your range and awareness of fuel percentages will become a very natural part of the decisions you make about your meals.

As for Principle No. 2, I hope I've convinced you that eating at least five meals a day is not only a requirement for weight loss and management but is also the most satisfying and healthy way to eat. Now that you know about the insulin response created with every meal, it should be easy as well as logical to stick to this natural eating pattern. The pay off is: minimizing hunger, stabilizing insulin levels, improving metabolism, promoting better health, and feeling and looking great!

Principle No. 3, what to eat, also supports an individualized program; you will plan your meals based on your personal preferences using the BOK Six Fuel Groups on the web site [icon] as your guide. You can plan for the week, day-by-day, or from one meal to the next. The primary principle is that you focus on the kind of fuel to eat, then make your food and meal choices accordingly. Get creative—your choices are almost limitless.

You can be just as creative with your exercise plan—there are so many options to choose from. You can stick to one program or change it up a little to reshape specific areas of your body. I suspect that some of you may still be resistant to the idea of resistance training. The idea of using free weights or exercise machines may be daunting if you've never used them before, especially if you feel self-conscious or awkward about exercising in public. But remember that you don't have to go to a gym or health club. There are many ways to incorporate resistance training into a home workout too. A set of light hand weights is all you need to get started, and focus on the Three Principles of Exercise: repetitions, technique, and breathing. Then choose from a list of activities and exercises on the web site [icon] and try out one of the weekly BOK 123 – ABC Exercise Plans. Many of my patients, particularly women, have told me that resistance training is enjoyable and rewarding. Your body will respond quickly if you stick to the BOK Switch Training technique, and seeing and feeling results is the ultimate motivator. As for aerobic exercise, I hope that I have convinced you just how easy it is to turn on the fat burner. Remember, if it makes you really huff and puff, then you are working too hard and are not burning fat. When you are working at your target heart rate, you should be able to maintain your pace for some time and burn fat more efficiently. You don't need to make it hard on yourself. Easy does it, and make it something you enjoy.

Designing Your Diet and Exercise Plan

Although the focus of Body of Knowledge is to empower you to create your own personalized programs, starting with a blank slate may seem overwhelming at first. To get you started, I've created five places to start, with general eating and exercise plans based on the most common patient archetypes that I have seen over the years in my clinics.

- **BOK – Troubles Around the Equator**™: For those of you who want to lose those extra layers around your midsection permanently.
- **BOK – Quick Fix**™: For those of you who want to slim down faster for an important life event.
- **BOK – Obesity**™: A safer, medically supervised program for those of you who need to lose a substantial amount of weight.
- **BOK – Alive, Well, and Feeling Great**™: For those of you who want to focus on better health, fitness, and longevity.
- **BOK – Too Thin**™: For those of you who want a healthy boost in size, strength, and vitality.

The BOKsystem is a *complete* weight-management system, so we have designed the first three plans for healthy weight loss, the fourth for weight maintenance, and the fifth for weight gain. Pick the plan that best applies to your present physical situation or desired goals and use it as a kick-off point to designing your own program. I suggest that you take a look at all of the plans because you may find a little bit of yourself in more than one of them. And if you don't already have a specific goal in mind, reading the goals for these plans may help you clarify yours—they all include healthy eating and exercise habits. You can also select one of these plans on the web site [icon] that already have sample exercises and meals included. Print them out, try them out, then add, delete, or change things up as you see fit.

It's time to take your new knowledge and put it to work!

BOK – Troubles Around the Equator

Call it portly or pear-shaped; call them love-handles, saddlebags, or a beer belly—by any name, the accumulation of fat around our midsections is the most ubiquitous weight problem today. I believe that it represents everything that is wrong with the American lifestyle: poor eating habits, unhealthy food choices, and lack of exercise. But fear not; the baggage you carry up front, around your hips, and on your backside can all be eliminated.

Food Choices

First and foremost are your eating habits. But don't worry about starving. Meal frequency (Principle No. 2) is mandatory for fat loss no matter where it sits. Five to seven meals a day should be your foundation. As for calorie reduction, I recommend that you take it slow in order to lose those layers and keep them off.

If you exercise in the morning, follow the guidelines for the BOK Fat Loss / Weight Maintenance Meal Plan and the 2:1 carb-to-protein ratio for meals one and two. Then, depending upon your energy needs, switch to the BOK Accelerated Fat Loss Meal Plan and the 1:1 carb-to-protein ratio to finish out your day.

All exercise (especially resistance training) requires more carbs, so the meal preceding your workout should have at least the 2:1 carb-to-protein ratio.

Because so much fat is centered in one place, you should be able to feel results in a few weeks and start seeing results in a few months. And once you see results, I encourage you to step it up a bit.

Principle No. 3, what to eat, offers you a lot of flexibility in battling the bulge. Concentrate your food choices on fuel groups 1, 2, and 3 (unprocessed) and go easy on the higher fat foods found in groups 4, 5, and 6. It's important to reduce your fat intake, but it is unrealistic and unhealthy to go completely fat free. For best results, stick with small amounts of quality unsaturated fats and try to avoid group 6 altogether. You most likely got into trouble around your equator because of a fondness for processed foods. You need to find a way to stay away from them. I do realize that many of these Fat Cocktail foods may be old comforting friends, and it may be difficult to cut them out entirely. If you can't go cold turkey, wean yourself off of processed foods at a comfortable pace and try to eat them in the meal before or close to your workout but never before bedtime. You can overcome your cravings for them—in fact, you will—just stay focused on your new mental clarity and physical changes that the BOK Three Principles will produce. There is also more knowledge to come in Part 5, Mind Over Matter. We will address other obstacles that may prevent you from reaching your goals, but if you are not losing weight or are not seeing a shrinking waistline, it is a sign you need to first reevaluate your eating habits before you step up your exercise. Below is a quick meal strategy overview with two sample meals. You'll find the rest of this meal strategy as well as complete weekly meal strategies for all our plans on the BOK web site.

SAMPLE WEEKLY MEAL STRATEGY FOR BOK – TROUBLES AROUND THE EQUATOR

Principle No. 2 How Often to Eat (Minimum 5 meals)	Principle No. 1 How Much to Eat (% of daily calories carb-to-protein-to-fat ratio)	Principle No. 3 What to Eat (Carb, protein, and fat quality)	Rationale
Meal 1: Breakfast	10% of daily calories 60:30:10 gram ratio	2:1 carb-to-protein ratio Carbs: Simple allowed, complex mix optimal Protein: Lean Fat: Suggested ratio	Carbs in the morning are needed to give you your first energy boost of the day. If you crave simple carbs, this is the time to eat them because you are less likely to store them—you have all day to burn them.
Meal 2: Morning Snack	15% of daily calories 60:30:10 gram ratio	2:1 carb-to-protein ratio Carbs: Simple and complex mix Protein: Lean Fat: Suggested ratio	Start to lean toward complex carbs, but simple carbs are still allowed because of your energy needs, especially if you exercise before or after breakfast.

*full version available on the website

Exercise

Exercise should consist of a weekly mix of aerobic and anaerobic activities. For best results, work on your thighs using a higher rep-etition BOK Switch Training program for toning, focus more on your abdominals, but don't forget to also focus on your upper body as well. This will offer a two-fold advantage. First, the extra muscle mass you acquire will improve your overall fat burning metabolism.

Second, building your upper body will develop and firm up an area of neglect and create a weight loss optical illusion.

Building up your upper body can make your lower body seem smaller by comparison (especially if your lower body is shrinking at the same time). If you're a man, you want to strive more for a V-shape. If you're a woman, it is probably best to strive for a balance between your upper and lower areas.

For those of you without major medical problems, I recommend starting with a slight variation of the BOK Exercise Plan 1-C and work your way up to the BOK Exercise Plan 2-C. Obviously a more extensive mix of BOK Switch Training combined with stricter eating habits will maximize your results and help you reach your goals in a shorter time period. You'll find a sample of 2-C below. The full plan is on the web site as well.

SAMPLE WEEKLY EXERCISE STRATEGY FOR BOK – TROUBLES AROUND THE EQUATOR

BOK EXERCISE PLAN 2-C:

- 4 days per week BOK Switch Training
- 4 days per week short aerobic exercise
- 1 day per week long aerobic exercise
- 2 days of rest

Day	Exercise	Weight	Sets	Repetition/ Duration
Monday	Upper Body BOK Switch Training Abdominals Short aerobic exercise	Moderate — —	2–3 2–3 —	8–15 reps 15–50 reps 15–20 minutes
Tuesday	Lower Body BOK Switch Training Abdominals Short aerobic exercise	Moderate — —	2–3 2–3 —	8–15 reps 15–50 reps 15–20 minutes

*full version available on the website

Extra Ammunition

One important issue to consider is alcohol consumption. This refined carbohydrate likes to stimulate fat accumulation at your equator. The infamous "beer belly" forms by combining the processed carbs from the distilling process and the sedentary aftermath that results from the disinhibition that alcohol creates. Alcohol also contains more calories than other carbs—seven calories per gram as compared to four. Wine and other liquors can contain even more sugar content than beer, but vodka, gin, bourbon, whiskey, scotch, and other "hard" alcohols, with or without mixers, can do the same damage. Fat production and storage at your midsection is accelerated by the concentration of these carbs absorbed through your intestinal tract. And the disinhibition or "buzz" that follows alcohol consumption customarily invites poor food choices (usually more simple carbs, fat, and salt) that add to the fat-friendly environment.

Lastly, suck in that gut! Posture is an important step in maintaining a flatter tummy. Once the abdominal muscles are stretched past your belt line, they do not contract or function properly. They are designed to stabilize your torso by contracting vertically, not with a circular arc. Concentrate on keeping your lower abs pulled inward when you are exercising them and maintain this posture as much as possible throughout the day.

BOK – Quick Fix

In my experience, most people who want to shed their final ten to twenty pounds fall into two categories: those who don't care about the extra weight until a special event turns on the motivation (class reunion or trip to the beach), and those who have reached a plateau in their weight loss. Whether you are ready to break that plateau, get into your tuxedo or fit into that special dress or bathing suit, you, like so many others, are ready to put in some extra effort to lose pounds fast. I'm here to tell you that it can be done—and done safely. All it takes is the focus and desire to follow this plan until you lose that extra size or those last few inches.

This is only a short-term plan, as it is very difficult to stick to it for any length of time. It is specifically designed to help you lose fat in a short period of time. It requires strict adherence to the BOK Accelerated Fat Loss Meal Plan and a modified exercise regimen. This plan is designed with the young and healthy in mind, so consult your doctor if you have any concerns.

Food Choices

Cutting calories is priority one in this plan. Reduce your daily calorie intake by 20 percent as explained in the description of the BOK Accelerated Fat Loss Meal Plan, then go to the web site, which is where you can find the complete BOK – Quick Fix meal strategy. You can cut calories a bit more as long as you can function well, mentally and physically, throughout the day. Equally important is adhering to the 1:1 carb-to-protein ratio, as well as minimizing fat in all of your meals. Lastly, try to avoid all processed carbohydrates, select more complex, unprocessed carbohydrates (especially as the day progresses), eat lean protein only, and stick with the unsaturated varieties of fats in the foods you select.

SAMPLE WEEKLY MEAL STRATEGY FOR BOK – QUICK FIX

Principle No. 2 How Often to Eat (6 meals)	Principle No. 1 How Much to Eat (% of daily calories carb-to-protein-to-fat ratio)	Principle No. 3 What to Eat (Carb, protein, and fat quality)	Rationale
Meal 1: Breakfast	10% of daily calories 45:45:*10 gram ratio	1:1 carb-to-protein ratio Carbs: Unprocessed only, restrict simple to fruit Protein: Lean, no specifics Fat: Suggested ratio	A small carb and protein meal mix is good in the morning to minimize an early surge of insulin. Limit simple carbs to fruit.
Meal 2: Morning Snack	15% of daily calories 45:45:*10 gram ratio	1:1 carb-to-protein ratio Carbs: Complex, restrict simple to fruit Protein: Lean only Fat: Suggested ratio	Simple carbs and foods that contain more fat earlier in the day are better especially if exercise is performed at this time.

*full version available on the website

Exercise

The exercise regimen for this plan is also rigid but simple: do as much aerobic activity as you can handle without risking injury or overuse syndromes. This is a great way to keep your metabolism revved up and temporarily suppress hunger. I recommend a minimum of aerobic activity four days a week, but five to six days with one or two days of light exercise and one day of rest will take off the pounds at the fastest rate. Also don't forget to drink water—enough to meet the standards given in the BOK Ten Essential Tips for Weight Management. Below is a sample version of the BOK Exercise Plan 3-A, altered for quick weight loss with just enough BOK Switch Training to maintain muscle mass and the ability to vary your aerobic exercises. The full plan can be found on the web site, ready for customization. You may notice that all the rules of muscle development and maintenance are absent here, but truthfully they may go against your goals on this short-term plan if shrinking your waist or fitting into particular clothing are your priorities. Keeping your muscle mass at its present size or having just a little bit of atrophy (muscle loss) may help these goals and give you your best results. While fat loss is a priority for you right now, don't put it before your health and sanity. It's not worth it. Take it down a notch or consult your doctor if you feel any adverse physical or mental effects during this period.

SAMPLE WEEKLY EXERCISE STRATEGY FOR BOK – QUICK FIX

BOK EXERCISE PLAN 3-A:

- 2 days per week BOK Switch Training
- 2 days per week short aerobic exercise
- 4 days per week long aerobic exercise
- 1 day of rest

Day	Type of Exercise	Weight	Sets	Repetitions/Duration
Monday	Total body BOK Switch Training	Moderate	1	8–15 reps
	Abdominals	—	1	15–50 reps
	Short aerobic exercise	—	—	20–30 minutes
Tuesday	Long aerobic exercise	—	—	30–60 minutes
	Abdominals	—	1	15–50 reps

*full version available on the website

BOK – Obesity

Most people who are moderately or severely overweight have been struggling with this problem all of their lives. No matter what program they select or how hard they try, the weight they lose usually comes right back—often more weight than what they lost. It leads to a vicious cycle of gaining, losing, and gaining even more. Sadly, the end result is often a diagnosis of clinical obesity, meaning a person with a body mass index (BMI) of 30 or higher. I encourage you to go to the web site to find your body mass index and learn more about obesity.

For medical professionals, making the decision to recommend a diet and exercise program is not easy, so we use the BMI and waist circumference guide as a screening tool and then perform a complete history and physical evaluation before giving a patient the nod to start on their program. More and more studies have focused on the relationship between BMI, waist circumference, and the risk of disease, as indicated in the table on the next page. The most important consideration for substantial weight loss is medical supervision throughout the program before, during, and after you have achieved your goals. Anyone fighting obesity, especially those with health problems, will need a medical evaluation and constant supervision until their doctor advises otherwise. Serious weight problems are frequently rooted in issues that require professional counseling too. I highly recommend that my obese patients undergo some type of initial screening and counseling (which they will hopefully continue throughout the duration of the program) to help them identify habits that contribute to

173

their problems with weight management and find ways to neutralize their influence.

CHILDHOOD OBESITY: A NATIONAL EPIDEMIC

It could be a weed in your lawn, a little white lie, or a viral outbreak.

Or, it could be a child starting life with a weight problem. If you don't stop it early, it is a problem that can grow out of control. In fact, it already has.

Childhood obesity is approaching epidemic proportions. Obesity in children ages six to eleven has doubled in the last twenty years and is now at an all-time high. Obesity in adolescents ages twelve to nineteen has tripled. In fact, one out of five children in the United States is obese. And that is just for obesity—being 20 percent or more over the appropriate weight for age and height. The statistics on children who are "only" overweight are even more alarming! Read the full article, "Can Love Be Fattening?" on the web site [icon] and find out more about the causes and solutions to this national epidemic in "Divine Intervention."

Finding the psychological origin of the eating and health habits that bring people to obese weight levels is the only way to solve the problem permanently. If you are clinically obese, it is essential that you read Part 5. Unless you resolve your underlying issues, you are more likely to keep regaining any weight you may lose. One important point to remember is that it will take a little time (several months at least) for severely obese people (BMI greater than 35) to really notice any changes in the way they feel or look.

Lastly, be honest with yourself. Depending upon the amount of weight that needs to be lost and the level of fitness gained, it can take up to a year to reach your goals. If a healthy rate of weight loss is two pounds a week, then that's what it will take to lose one hundred pounds. Try to remain focused, realistic, and patient. If you find yourself frustrated, keep in mind that the pounds you are shedding are still coming off much faster than the time it took to put them on. Now you have both time and your new knowledge on your side.

WEIGHT CLASSIFICATION, BMI, WAIST CIRCUMFERENCE, AND ASSOCIATED DISEASE RISK

Disease Risk* Relative to Normal Weight and Waist Circumference

	BMI (kg/m2)	Class	Men ≤102 cm (≤ 40 in) / Women ≤88 cm (≤35 in)	>102 cm (>40 in) / >88 cm (>35 in
Underweight	<18.5		—	—
Normal†	18.5–24.9		—	—
Overweight	25.0–29.9		Increased	High
Obesity	30.0–34.9	I	High	Very High
	35.0–39.9	II	Very High	Very High
Extreme Obesity	≥40	III	Extremely High	Extremely High

* Disease risk for type 2 diabetes, hypertension, and cardiovascular disease.

† Increased waist circumference can also be a marker for increased risk even in persons of normal weight. Source: Adapted from "Obesity: Preventing and Managing the Global Epidemic." Report of the World Health Organization Consultation of Obesity. WHO, Geneva, June 1997. As referenced in "Clinical Guidelines on the Identification, Evaluation, and Treatment of Overweight and Obesity in Adults." *The Evidence Report*, September 1998. NIH Publication: National Institute of Health, National Heart, Lung and Blood Institute in cooperation with The National Institute of Diabetes and Digestive and Kidney Diseases.

Food Choices

If you are obese or extremely obese, a change in diet must be your number one priority. Since your eating habits have most likely been in place for a long time, I recommend a gradual change. Major calorie restriction is dangerous and can not only aggravate or create adverse medical conditions but also the "gain, lose, gain more" cycle we discussed earlier. In terms of total daily calories, people who are obese and extremely obese should maintain a comfortable level of caloric intake for the first month of the new program. Principle No. 2, eating frequency and eating smaller meals (five to seven per day), is your starting top priority. Set your watch, your alarm clock, mobile phone, or find someone to join you in the buddy system. Just make this happen because it is your only chance to eat less without a surgical procedure. Changing the quality of your meals should also begin right away. Try to stick with unprocessed foods from fuel groups 1, 2, and 3. Keep foods from groups 4 and 5 to a minimum and try to avoid all foods from group 6 entirely. Then reward yourself once a week with a few of the old comfort foods if you haven't overcome your cravings.

After a few months of strict adherence to Principles No. 2 and No. 3, turn your attention to Principle No. 1, size of meals. Initially, try removing 250 to 500 calories a day from your total daily calories. Stay at this level for three to six months, then remove another 100 to 200 daily calories each month until you end up at your recommended daily caloric intake for your age, gender, height, and weight goal. If you are handling the change well, both physically and mentally, and you want faster results, you can try the BOK Accelerated Fat Loss Meal Plan guidelines and speed things up a bit. Just continue to stay in close contact with your primary care physician or obesity specialist and alert them to any changes first. The complete sample weekly five meal strategy, ready to be customized according to your personal needs, can be found on the web site.

SAMPLE WEEKLY MEAL STRATEGY FOR BOK – OBESITY

Principle No. 2 How Often to Eat (6 meals)	Principle No. 1 How Much to Eat (% of daily calories carb-to-protein-to-fat ratio)	Principle No. 3 What to Eat (Carb, protein, and fat quality)	Rationale
Meal 1: Breakfast	10% of daily calories 60:30:10 gram ratio	2:1 carb-to-protein ratio Carbs: Simple allowed, complex mix optimal Protein: Lean Fat: Maximize unsaturated, minimize saturated	Carbs in the morning are needed to give you your first energy boost of the day. If you crave simple carbs, this is the time to eat them because you are less likely to store them—you have all day to burn them.
Meal 2: Morning Snack	15% of daily calories 60:30:10 gram ratio	2:1 carb-to-protein ratio Carbs: Simple and complex mix Protein: Lean Fat: Maximize unsaturated, minimize saturated	Start to lean toward complex carbs, but simple carbs are still allowed because of your energy needs, especially if you exercise before or after breakfast.

*full version available on the website

Exercise

Sometimes, because of health status and stature, exercise is not an option for people who are obese. If you fall into this category, again you should consult your primary care physician or obesity specialist first. For example, a physical examination, specific blood tests, or even cardiac stress testing may be necessary before even the most rudimentary exercise is begun. Those people who have a BMI greater than 30, have had some type of musculoskeletal impairment, or are under a doctor's care for a medical condition need to get clearance from their doctor before undertaking any exercise program, even a mild, beginner-oriented one.

Phase I: Muscle Education

The early phase of your exercise program should be directed toward muscle education and cardiovascular stimulation. Like the change in your eating habits, this phase should last for at least two to three months to give your heart and lungs time to acclimate to the change, to make progress in your range of motion, and to minimize other problems, such as fatigue, soreness, and cramping. Examples include water aerobics, stationary bicycling, and other non-impact calisthenics approved by your doctor or a certified trainer who is experienced with obese clients. Complete examples for Phase I, II and III samples can be found on the web site.

Sample Phase I Weekly Exercise Strategy for BOK – Obesity

Day	Exercise	Weight	Sets	Duration
Monday	Stretching	—	1	5 minutes per muscle group
Tuesday	*Aerobic exercise with extremity ROM	—	—	15–30 minutes

*full version available on the website

**Type, duration, and frequency of aerobic exercise approved by your doctor.

Phase II: Muscle Toning

After a few months, your phase I activities should become effortless (and possibly boring) so build on your success by changing your workout program to promote more muscle tone. Remember that increased muscle tone will improve your strength and metabolism. High repetition resistance training will tone your muscles and also improve your coordination. Machines at a health club or small hand weights at home are a great place to start. You can start by choosing a program from

BOK Exercise Plans 1 (A, B, or C) that fits your lifestyle. Concentrate on your breathing and your technique to build a solid foundation and to avoid developing bad habits that can cause undue stress or injury. With your new eating habits and toned muscles, you now have the essential tools to reach your goals at a healthy pace.

SAMPLE PHASE II WEEKLY EXERCISE STRATEGY FOR BOK – OBESITY

BOK EXERCISE PLAN 1-A:

- 2 days per week BOK Switch Training
- 2 days per week short aerobic exercise
- 2 days per week long aerobic exercise
- 3 days of rest

Day	Type of Exercise	Weight	Sets	Repetitions/ Duration
Monday	Total body Switch Training	Light	1	10–12 reps
	Abdominals	—	1	15–50 reps
	Short aerobic exercise	—	—	15–20 minutes
Tuesday	Rest			

*full version available on the website

Phase III: Muscle Development

Phase III is an optional plan for those who want to develop their muscles beyond the toning phase. Even if you are younger or have a clean bill of health, I recommend that you do not step up to this level of exercise until you are closer to your target weight (or healthier lean-to-fat mass ratio) and can perform proper techniques for all of the toning exercises you have chosen. In Phase II you worked on increasing the tone and strength of your body core and extremities. Now your muscles are ready for more resistance and further development. Lower your re petitions (but no fewer than ten or twelve reps) and try to increase the amount of weight to a level that feels comfortable. Your goal is to gain strength and lean mass slowly, so aim for a "tight" or slightly sore feeling for one to three days after a workout in the beginning. That feeling is your body getting ready for its next session, so wait until it passes (or follow the three to four day recovery rule) before you exercise the same muscle groups again.

As for your aerobic exercise and rest days, they are interchangeable, and you can vary your activity on those days as your schedule changes. If you are performing the recommended BOK Switch Training, you are already getting some aerobic conditioning. Choose any level in the BOK Exercise Plans 2 (A, B, or C) that is comfortable both physically and mentally. Below is a modified, introductory version of the BOK Exercise Plan 2-C using light to moderate weight and only one set per muscle group. Eventually you can increase your sets, try new techniques, weights, machines, and aerobic activities and reschedule your week accordingly until you reach your particular goals. My goal for you is to make exercise feel good and to make it a part of your life like any other important priority.

Sample Phase III Weekly Exercise Strategy for BOK – Obesity

BOK Exercise Plan 2-C:

- 4 days per week BOK Switch Training
- 4 days per week short aerobic exercise
- 1 day per week long aerobic exercise
- 2 days of rest

Day	Type of Exercise	Weight	Sets	Repetitions/ Duration
Monday	Upper body Switch Training	Light to moderate	1	10–15 reps
	Abdominals	—	1	15–50 reps
	Short aerobic exercise	—	—	15–20 mins
Tuesday	Lower body Switch Training	Light to moderate	1	10–15 reps
	Abdominals	—	1	15–50 reps
	Short aerobic exercise	—	—	15–20 mins

*full version available on the website

BOK – Alive, Well, and Feeling Great

Right now, you have it all: you feel great, you look great, and you're as happy as a fit person can be. All you can ask for is that your good health and happiness continue throughout your lifetime. Or maybe you are one of those people who looks good but you've put your health on the line living in the fast lane? Or maybe you're dealing with the effects of a medical condition but still look and feel okay. Or maybe you simply have concerns about getting older. Whatever your situation, you are now making a conscious decision to get the best out of life. This is what the BOK Fat Loss / Weight Maintenance Meal Plan is all about.

Food Choices

This plan is designed to help you develop good habits that focus on eating unprocessed foods, eating five to seven meals a day, and maintaining smaller healthy portions.

Try to choose vegetables and fruits for the majority of your carbs, lean meats for the majority of your protein and nuts for the majority of your fats. Drink plenty of water and minimize your sodium intake. The goal is to supply your machine with the right fuels throughout the day, providing it with all of the natural vitamins and minerals necessary to accommodate its original design. Let's turn back the hands of time before manufacturers started messing around with food in the name of convenience. You can find the entire week sample on the web site, as well as other customizable meal strategies to fit your lifestyle.

SAMPLE WEEKLY MEAL STRATEGY FOR BOK – ALIVE, WELL AND FEELING GREAT

Principle No. 2 How Often to Eat (Minimum 5 meals)	Principle No. 1 How Much to Eat (% of daily calories carb-to-protein-to-fat ratio)	Principle No. 3 What to Eat (Carb, protein, and fat quality)	Rationale
Meal 1: Breakfast	10% of daily calories 60:30:10 gram ratio	2:1 carb-to-protein ratio Carbs: Simple okay Protein: Lean, no specifics Fat: Maximize unsaturated, limit saturated	A small meal is best with a mix of all three fuels. You are less likely to store simple carbs because of a greater energy expenditure with normal morning activities.
Meal 2: Morning Snack	15% of daily calories 60:30:10 gram ratio	2:1 carb-to-protein ratio Carbs: Simple and complex Protein: Lean, no specifics Fat: Maximize unsaturated, limit saturated	This meal should be the same size as or slightly larger than your breakfast. Simple carbs are okay, especially if exercising early or at lunchtime.

*full version available on the website

Exercise

The first plan's weekly exercise strategy involves more time exercising, but will help you maintain your physical results easier and allow for some additional development or sculpting too. If you feel that maintenance is your main goal, though, then I suggest you visit the BOK web site to see both weekly exercise strategies in their completion. They are a simple mix of muscle development and conditioning and will bring you to a point of optimum health—and keep you there.

Two Sample Weekly Exercise Strategies for BOK – Alive, Well, and Feeling Great

Example I: Resistance Training Four Times a Week

This is a good choice for those who want to maintain their results easily. If life gets in the way of your workouts from time to time, it will quickly get you back on track. It also has the potential for continued development if you stay focused, and it flows nicely with a traditional five-day work week. Your sets are variable and depend upon your goals and time constraints. The extended aerobic exercise days are optional and give you the option of better endurance or more fat loss. They could be substituted for rest days, depending upon time constraints or fatigue. You can find the full example for this plan and Example II: Resistance Training Twice a Week on the web site. 📖

BOK EXERCISE PLAN 2-C:

- 4 days per week BOK Switch Training
- 4 days per week short aerobic exercise
- 1 day per week long aerobic exercise
- 2 days of rest

Day	Exercise	Weight	Sets	Repetitions/ Duration
Monday	Upper body Switch Training Abdominals Short aerobic exercise	Moderate — —	1–3 2–3 —	8–15 reps 15–50 reps 15–20 mins
Tuesday	Lower body Switch Training Abdominals Short aerobic exercise	Moderate — —	1–3 2–3 —	8–15 reps 15–50 reps 15–20 mins

*full version available on the website

Example II: Resistance Training Twice a Week

Resistance training twice a week is a popular regimen for people with time constraints. If you pay close attention to your eating habits, you can still maintain your muscle mass and remain injury free with only two resistance training sessions per week. Try to keep the sessions three to four days apart and bump up the intensity during these two workouts if you want to maintain similar results as training three to four times a week.

BOK EXERCISE PLAN 3-A:

- 2 days per week BOK Switch Training
- 2 days per week short aerobic exercise
- 4 days per week long aerobic exercise
- 1 day of rest

Day	Exercise	Weight	Sets	Repetitions/ Duration
Monday	Total body Switch Training Abdominals Short aerobic exercise	Moderate — —	3–5 2–3 —	8–15 reps 15–50 reps 20–30 minutes
Tuesday	Long aerobic exercise Abdominals	— —	— 2–3	30–60 minutes 15–50 reps

*full version available on the website

BOK – Too Thin

There is thin and there is too thin. And then there is scrawny. Barney Fife and Olive Oyl look-alikes can be just as sensitive about their body images as those carrying excess baggage. Gangly teenage boys can feel social pressure to bulk up, with or without the need to develop size for particular sports. An athletic build with muscle definition has traditionally been the goal of most young men, but today it is also one for many women. Having more lean muscle mass also promotes good health and longevity. And let's face it: a lean, muscular frame is attractive. It pleases me to no end to see men working for smaller, fitter frames and women sporting sleeveless shirts that display their toned biceps.

Then there are those who are thin for reasons other than their ectomorph body type. Social pressures to be very thin can come from many sources, and some people fall prey to eating disorders such as anorexia and bulimia. We will examine these sources in Part 5. And for some people, a medical condition or disease, such as cancer or AIDS, has resulted in weight loss or malnutrition. For the very thin, gaining weight can be just as difficult as it is for the overweight to lose it. Regardless of the cause, the first priority is to build and maintain a healthy level of muscle mass. And a healthy amount of dietary fat is necessary to keep it around and promote good health. Even for those with other medical conditions or diseases, a healthy diet and exercise program are just as important for healing and recovery as the best traditional medical treatments available.

Food Choices

So what should you eat? You would think that adding foods that contain the Fat Cocktail is all that would be needed to throw on a few pounds, but not so. The fat, salt, sugar combination does not contribute to the most important part of gaining healthy weight: more lean mass derived from healthy building blocks. A variety of meats and plant protein as well as sufficient carbohydrate and fat calories are the keys to adding healthy weight. Unprocessed foods will provide the essential vitamins and minerals to support proper growth and good health. I recommend a mix of complex and simple carbs for most meals. Use a 3:1 simple-carb-to-protein ratio after resistance training until your muscle mass reaches a healthy level. Fats can vary, but try not to slip below a percentage of 20 to 30 percent gram weight until you see a steady weight gain or are confident that your results aren't slipping away. For healthy individuals, I recommend that you should not go beyond a range of 35 to 45 percent fat (still in gram weight), but consult your doctor first since certain individuals or specific medical conditions can have adverse reactions to a high fat diet. As for the quality, some saturated fat from meat, dairy, and eggs is fine, but the plant and nut oils should be your mainstay, as well as fat from animal protein high in omega-3 fatty acids.

It may seem like a no-brainer to just eat more, but here's how to do it intelligently. An extra 500 calories a day (up to or past your target daily calories) should add up to a healthy one-pound-a-week increase. If you aren't gaining at this rate, try to add more carbs to your post-workout meal and your meal before bedtime (still at least one and a half hours before you hit the sack). Meal frequency is also flexible. You have to determine what works best for you. I recommend three to four larger meals a day rather than the usual five to seven so that your insulin levels jump a little higher after each meal and increase your storage capacity. So if three squares a day with a big meal at night give you the best results, go with it until you reach your goal. Then you can add a meal and return to the standard BOK Fat Loss / Weight Maintenance Meal Plan to keep your results and avoid gaining too much. The key is to continue eating the right foods, accept slow and steady results, and pay as close attention to how you feel as you do to the mirror and the scale. The complete sample meal strategy can be found on the web site.

	SAMPLE WEEKLY MEAL STRATEGY FOR BOK – TOO THIN		
Principle No. 2 How Often to Eat (Minimum 5 meals)	**Principle No. 1** How Much to Eat (% of daily calories carb-to-protein-to-fat ratio	**Principle No. 3** What to Eat (Carb, protein, and fat quality)	**Rationale**
Meal 1: Breakfast	15% of daily calories 50:25:*25 gram ratio	2:1 carb-to-protein ratio Carbs: Simple Protein: No specifics Fat: Mix of saturated and unsaturated	It is best to have a large meal with simple carbs, protein and fat early to boost insulin levels to maximize muscle building and development, particularly if exercising before or after breakfast.
Meal 2: Lunch	30% of daily calories 50:25:*25 gram ratio	2:1 carb-to-protein ratio Carbs: Simple and complex Protein: No specifics Fat: Mix of saturated and unsaturated	Mixing complex and unprocessed carbs with simple carbs ensures proper nutrition, health and muscle maintenance.

*Fat percentages can vary, but do not go beyond 30–45%.
**full version available on the website

187

Exercise

As for exercise, you will obviously concentrate on resistance training to build more muscle mass. Fewer repetitions and more weight has always been a great formula for this, and BOK Switch Training is a better technique to make the most of your efforts. If you are an exercise novice, start with a toning program for muscle coordination and education. Then increase your weight as your strength and size develop.

The exercise strategy on the next page is part of an alteration of the BOK Exercise Plan 1-C that has no long aerobic exercise days. I also increased the amount of sets and decreased the amount of repetitions to give you the best chance to build and maintain healthy muscle mass. You can find the full version on the BOK web site. Of course other aerobic activities are not forbidden, but calories are calories, and burning too many of them will go against your goals early in the game. Once you have reached your resistance training goals, you can add aerobic exercise to your program, but initially it should not go beyond thirty minutes. The "twitch" muscle cells we discuss on the web site, developed from conditioning exercises, will compete with and compromise the ones (strength and size) you develop from weight training. And don't forget that BOK Switch Training performed correctly has an inherent aerobic component. Just try to keep your extra aerobic activity in the recreational category. Ride bikes with your children or take a walk, but keep your focus on weight training and allow your muscle groups enough time to rest between workouts to heal and maximize development.

SAMPLE WEEKLY EXERCISE STRATEGIES FOR BOK – TOO THIN

BOK EXERCISE PLAN 1-C:

- 4 days per week Switch Training
- 4 days per week short aerobic exercise
- 3 days of rest

Day	Exercise	Weight	Sets	Repetitions/ Duration
Monday	Upper body Switch Training Abdominals Short aerobic exercise	Moderate — —	1–3 2–3 —	8–15 reps 15–50 reps 15–20 minutes
Tuesday	Lower body Switch Training Abdominals Short aerobic exercise	Moderate — —	1–3 2–3 —	8–15 reps 15–50 reps 15–20 minutes

*full version available on the website

Keep Your Shape and Your Sanity

Just a few things to keep in mind for maintaining your hard-earned results. The Body of Knowledge program that you have developed for yourself is more than enough ammunition to help you maintain your success.

The best strategy to keep your shape and sanity is to combine the BOK Meal and Exercise Plans that are working for you with the additional knowledge you have gained and to continue to monitor any changes your body may be experiencing so that you can adjust your program accordingly. The only thing we haven't discussed yet are common physical side effects that get in the way of your workouts and can make you want give up, like stiffness, soreness, muscle burning, fatigue, or even fitness plateaus. We will show you how to work through or around them in the next section, Mind Over Matter.

But there may come a time when you are at or close to your goals and need to notch it down a bit. If you have important projects that take you away from your routine for an extended amount of time, find yourself in a family crisis, or just want to take a break from the health club to do nothing other than relax on a two week vacation, just refocus your efforts on time management and efficiency. Remember, food quality and quantity are the strongest influences on your hard-earned results, but a few simple exercises at home, work, or while traveling can minimize muscle atrophy and maintain your muscle memory.

No doubt, the same Body of Knowledge that got you in good shape and good health can help you get back. But there are obstacles other than the physical ones I mentioned. You may find that these predictable and unpredictable life events let stress, worry, anxiety, depression, and other issues get in your way too. They are nothing to be ashamed of and should never be ignored. Understanding these mental obstacles and the physical barriers they create is a major part of your overall strategy for success.

Let's move on to Part 5, Mind Over Matter, expose some old myths, learn how simple it is to avoid or overcome some of these obstacles, explore some of the more serious problems, and put the finishing touches on your Body of Knowledge.

PART 5

MIND OVER MATTER

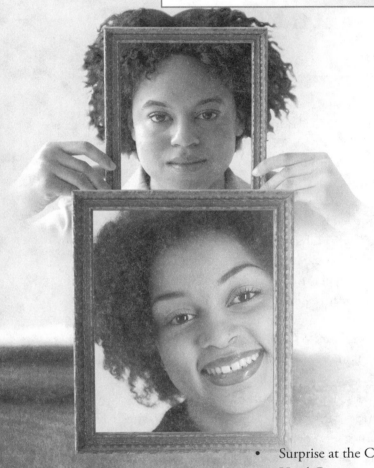

Surprise at the Clinic

Tracy got off of the scale with a shy grin. She walked quietly into the room and sat down. "Tracy has now lost forty-eight pounds, everyone!" I reported proudly to the rest of the group in the weight-management program. Her cheeks were flushed red, and her smile revealed her joy as she fought back tears.

I, too, was moved because I had grown fond of her three-year-old daughter, Debby, who often accompanied her to our weekly group sessions. I saw Tracy's new healthy lifestyle as a chance for Debby to avoid the weight problems that had a long history in Tracy's family. Tracy would be a great role model, I thought.

Tracy not only continued to lose more and more weight as the weeks went by, she also lowered her cholesterol and blood pressure enough to stop taking medications. Tracy was a living example of everything I had hoped to give people through my Body of Knowledge plans. And as pleased as I was with her physical progress, I was also pleased to see her positive attitude and growing self-esteem. Eventually she lost another seventy pounds and became a mentor for some of the new patients. Her health and happiness were an inspiration.

One day I caught myself gazing at her daughter with pride as she clung to her mother's slim, energetic body. They looked so happy. I thought my job was done.

I was wrong.

The truth of the matter was that I had only assisted Tracy with half of her problem. The other half still lay dormant. Lurking behind the bright eyes and positive attitude was a growing tension no one could have imagined. Eventually, she stopped coming to the clinic, but I assumed she was enjoying her new way of life and had decided to close the door on the past. Then, a few years later she showed up at my surgical practice with an ankle problem. I couldn't believe my eyes. She had gained most of her weight back—close to a hundred pounds! And her positive, joyful attitude had disappeared. In fact, she was taking antidepressants. When I asked her what happened, she gave me an answer that shocks me to this day.

She said she never got used to living in her new body. It made her "uncomfortable." It wasn't too long before her initial happiness started to wane. She became so unhappy that she went back to her old habits and started to regain weight. Her disappointment, feelings of failure, and low self-esteem led to stress, anxiety, and eventually depression. She sought help with her primary care physician, who put her on antidepressants and suggested counseling.

I was incredulous. My first reaction was, "You've got to be kidding!"

Her shockingly honest reply was, "It's just easier this way."

Still lost, I rationalized that Tracy simply found it too hard to change her lifestyle permanently. But in reality, Tracy's weight management had little to do with what she ate, how often she exercised, or anything related to her body. Instead it had everything to do with her mind.

First she told me that it had made her extremely uncomfortable when men and women noticed her new physique. She felt people were "checking her out." Then she really pulled the rug out from under me, telling me "After I lost all that weight, my husband and I fought constantly. We finally started sleeping in separate beds."

Like most scientists, my confusion centered only on how illogical this all sounded. How could a slim body, good health, more energy, and renewed self-esteem cause this kind of misery for her and her family? It turns out that her outward exuberance a year prior was all a facade. The support and nurturing she received at the clinic ended the moment she walked out the door. She felt sabotaged in all other areas of her life, including her workplace and even at the community college she was attending. With her new, slimmer figure, offerings of cookies, candy, and other unhealthy snacks actually increased combined with comments like "Try one of these, Tracy. You can afford to eat them now."

Worst of all, she had absolutely no support system at home, the place where it was needed the most. It turns out that neither her husband nor her daughter appreciated what she had accomplished. In fact, they let it be known that they did not like the change and were happier with her being overweight—it represented the "real Tracy," the only person they had ever known.

But she *had* lost a lot of weight and appeared to be pleased with her results. They *must* have encouraged her in some way for her to have accomplished what she did. Not so. She said they did not help or support her in any way and that making the change was something she had done all by herself. I asked her if her husband and daughter would have helped if she asked them. She was quiet for a few moments then finally said, "They love me enough to help if I asked, but I know they really can't."

She continued to offer even more disturbing information about her lifestyle and habits, which led me to believe that she would benefit from additional counseling. I asked her to see a colleague who specialized in eating disorders. She agreed.

She returned to my office for a follow-up visit a month later ten pounds lighter. I was happy to see the return of a little of her former enthusiasm. We must have spent forty-five minutes talking before my nurse interrupted and told me that other patients were stacking up in the waiting room. She explained that, mentally, being obese was a more comfortable way of life for her because it was the only way she and the others in her life knew how to interact with her. Supporting the family dysfunctions and "going with the flow" avoided stress. It provided her with a feeling of security and

> HOW COULD A SLIM BODY, MORE ENERGY, AND RENEWED SELF-ESTEEM CAUSE SO MUCH MISERY?

"purpose" as well. Not only that, she felt her family showed more affection and love for her when she was overweight. And it was true. For them, living with thin Tracy was like living with a stranger. And this new stranger was disrupting all of the old, comfortable family issues and their dysfunctional relationship with food. To make a long story short, through counseling Tracy and her family worked together to find out exactly when, where, and how these feelings came to be and how to deal with them. Tracy learned how she became enmeshed in family dysfunctions passed down from generation to generation. Food simply fed their dysfunctional cycles with its tasty highs and lows.

This story has a happy ending, but there are many more stories that don't. Even the strictest eating and exercise intentions cannot overcome the mental demons that are often at the root of weight management problems. If you don't uncover and face these issues, you will have a very difficult time making a permanent change in your lifestyle. I will provide more details on this later, but let's take a look at the big picture first.

Head Games

If diet and exercise are the tools to keep your machine working smoothly, then the mind is the tool shed that protects them from outside influences. Your thoughts and feelings can keep you optimistic and on track as you develop your healthy lifestyle, or they can sabotage you and send you right back into your old, less-desirable habits. Whether it's cravings, soreness, fatigue, plateaus, or deeper issues sabotaging your fitness goals, finding out why they occur and what can be done to minimize their presence will give you an advantage that you may have never had in the past. That's what Tracy did, and it is the only reason Tracy ended up a winner in the end.

It is important to remain focused and feel secure in the knowledge that your new weight management and fitness program will deliver countless advantages in terms of your overall health, physical appearance, general outlook, and mental health. One of the best rewards from a successful program is achieving a greater level of mental peace (or less mental turmoil), which I believe translates into happiness.

Keep in mind that your machine is unique. It requires personal knowledge and personal responsibility to function properly. Your mind has the ability to correct its errors. It's the very place where misperceptions and misunderstandings start, and it is the only place to end them, so let's put it to work.

The key to staying on track is to have a working plan to circumvent the inevitable roadblocks and setbacks you will encounter. But before we get into the facts behind these obstacles, here are a few things to keep in mind when you get sidetracked by head games.

198

Mental Energy

There is no doubt that an energy equilibrium, or balance, exists in the mind. At any point in time, you only have so much total energy available, be it physical or mental. Although mental energy lacks a value that we can describe (such as calories), stress, emotions, decision-making, communication, or just thinking uses up a certain amount of energy. If you learn to understand the different mental influences and redirect their power, you can correctly balance your energy.

Think of mental balance as a scale that tilts like a seesaw as you experience positive or negative influences. You should strive for equilibrium. Yes, you must even avoid extensive periods of pleasure and ecstasy. Most of us connect food and emotions, which can result in dramatic energy imbalance—from the ecstasy of eating in excess to the self-punishment of calorie restriction the next day or the stressful efforts to burn the extra calories off.

> EFFORT TO REACH A PEACEFUL EQUILIBRIUM IS THE ONLY WAY TO CORRECT BOTH POSITIVE AND NEGATIVE SWINGS OF THE EMOTIONAL PENDULUM.

Everything that goes up must come down. And after periods of great highs, we often experience great lows. Food is too often a cause or a perceived solution to emotional imbalances; from disappointment to celebration, a common human response is to head for the refrigerator. For many people, it is an emotional response that's out of control. Drastic mood swings cannot be corrected with overt compensation that swings you too far in the other direction either. A conscious effort to reach a peaceful equilibrium is the only way to correct both positive and negative swings of the emotional pendulum. If you are experiencing negative emotions, such as anger, fear, guilt, or shame, positive emotions can steer you away from the downward spiral, but only a true return to a peaceful, neutral emotional state will correct either side of the scale.

Expectations

Expectations are outcomes we have imagined or hoped for in regard to particular events or pursuits. Often we try to turn our future hopes and dreams into reality without first understanding what's happening in the present. Expectations can act either as catalysts or obstacles to your health and fitness goals. Obviously, unmet expectations will cause mental strife, and better-than-expected outcomes will make your day, often causing euphoria or delusional pleasure. Win or lose, neither of these temporary mental states will give you a healthy balance of mental energy.

No matter how much you want to believe fitness advice or promises that sound overly attractive, the outcome that ultimately results from your efforts is the only thing that is or ever will be real.

Expectations create an imagined scenario of success in our minds before anything has actually happened. If it sounds too good to be true, then it is. Unrealistic expectations are only fodder for disappointment.

I encourage you to use the true knowledge that you've gained (and continue to educate yourself) to develop realistic diet and exercise expectations based on your personal goals and abilities. Give yourself some room for error buffered by a little acceptance of things that are out of your control. Try to remove all potentially disappointing expectations from this area of your life.

> UNREALISTIC EXPECTATIONS ARE ONLY FODDER FOR DISAPPOINTMENT.

Acceptance and Control

In Parts 2, 3, and 4 I offered many examples on which to base your personal fitness goals. And while you map out your own Body of Knowledge program with your best intention of succeeding, it is important that you are mentally prepared for setbacks. Successful planning is a wonderful thing, but don't expect success every day. You will have good days and great days, but you will also have difficult days and days when unexpected events will ruin your plans altogether. There is no way to control these unexpected events in your life.

I am not suggesting that you passively accept every slump or setback that gets in your way. Just avoid setting goals for yourself that leave no room for error, or for the inevitability that something will get in the way from time to time.

Trying to control things that you may have little control over will build unrealistic expectations. The adage "Whatever you think you control really controls you" is true. And that leads to discouragement and failure. The best overall results are achieved by accepting an

> AVOID SETTING GOALS FOR YOURSELF THAT LEAVE NO ROOM FOR ERROR.

uncontrollable situation and then doing your best to minimize its undesired effects. Acceptance of life's little obstacles is the best approach. To achieve this I suggest redirecting your energy that feeds off of the negative mindset of control to a more positive mindset that runs on the best form of mental energy around: *focus*.

Focus

Focus puts your mind back in charge of your thoughts and your body. Focus supplies a steady flow of energy to your mental machine. It turns on the thought process, puts you back on course, and helps keep you moving in the right direction. Focus is a higher level of mental effort on a task to match the physical effort you are expending. The way I see it, if a goal is really important to you, it won't matter if it takes an hour, a day, a month, or a year to achieve it. You can attain any goal if you just focus on it.

Focus minimizes self-doubt and feelings of failure. Your focus will be on the goal, not the obstacles or setbacks along the way. Mental focus will circumvent the unrealistic expectations and lack of acceptance you usually inflict upon yourself. And it is a great alternative to strict discipline because it is flexible and adapts to the daily priority changes we experience in our lives.

> YOU CAN ATTAIN ANY GOAL IF YOU JUST FOCUS ON IT.

Sensible Discipline

A certain level of discipline is an important part of any fitness regimen, but most often it involves rules and regulations that cannot be upheld consistently on a daily basis. If you focus on your particular daily goals and influences you will develop a more realistic form of discipline, which I call sensible discipline.

Sensible discipline helps most when your daily regimen has been disrupted or an unexpected opportunity arises. It's a modified "go with the flow" approach that allows you to change your plans according to life's little mishaps and still achieve your goals. For example, the next time you're stuck in a nasty traffic jam on your way to the health club or the jogging trails and you feel your blood begin to boil, turn around and go home. So you don't exercise that day. So what! Do it another day when you were planning to rest or take advantage of shops close by and do some errands that day instead. If you allow these small aggravations and setbacks to get to you, it will only take away from your enjoyment of your exercise program and healthy diet. Just practice sensible discipline, be ready to accept the unexpected, and adjust your schedule accordingly.

Life will continue to catch you off guard and test you in many other ways. Let's say you find yourself in a situation where there are absolutely no healthy food choices available. Should you starve? Of course not. Make the best choice possible and

> PRACTICE SENSIBLE DISCIPLINE, BE READY TO ACCEPT THE UNEXPECTED.

eat healthier at your next meal. Or, if you are staring at a super tasty temptation, there's nothing wrong with giving in on occasion, just have a small portion. Tomorrow you can return to your program and try a little harder for a day or two afterward until you have corrected the calorie imbalance. A little indulgence once in a while won't hurt as long as you can readjust, get back on track, and continue to focus on your goals.

Monitored Mania

I believe in living life to the fullest. For me, having a good time is not only essential, but it can replenish a low level of mental energy almost as effectively as sleep. Eating, or should I say feasting, is often a part of those good times. A feast can either commemorate a joyous event or offer comfort in troubled times.

A night, a day, or even a week-end of celebrating is a normal, natural part of human behavior. Why fight it? Every culture since the dawn of man has a history of occasional behavioral decadence, particularly in regards to food. If it's a

> ISN'T IT NICE TO KNOW THAT... ACCEPTANCE CAN REPLACE... GUILT?

birthday or an ancient tribal celebration, it's in our blood to rejoice and enjoy. While it shouldn't be an everyday occurrence, a good time once a month, more or less, without really overdoing it can be really good for your psyche. It certainly gives balance to a rigid lifestyle. And if this human trait is indeed a part of our DNA, I believe that acceptance is our only weapon against the eventual failure of trying to maintain constant willpower against it.

As long as you are consistently willing to change, adapt, and compensate, you can bend the "rules" once in a while and still reach your goals. Isn't it nice to know that the good feeling of acceptance can replace the bad feeling of guilt? So start examining your expectations, level of acceptance, and focus. Incorporate sensible discipline in your life and sneak in some monitored mania. It will make you a winner in any head game.

Ammunition for Success

During my days as a doctor in residence, I would frequently work twelve-to-sixteen hour days. That didn't leave much time to exercise or stick to a healthy diet. I recall one day in particular when anything and everything that could go wrong did go wrong—Murphy's Law in full swing. If I had any idea what was ahead of me that day I would have slammed off the alarm at 5:30 a.m. and gone back to sleep.

The previous three months of hospital rotations and the holiday season had taken their toll on my body, but I was firm in my resolve to get back in shape. Having just gotten back to my fitness routine, I awoke one morning with stiffness in my lower back and hamstring muscles. As my car rolled onto the freeway, I didn't notice the nearby construction and picked up a nail in my front tire. Boom! The car heaved into the shoulder. January can be as hot and humid as any other month in Houston, and my air-conditioning was blasting even though it was barely 7:00 a.m. By the time I changed the tire, my muscles were warmed up and I was sweating through my clothes. Then back to the air conditioned car, and my hamstrings and lower back tightened up even more. Off to the hospital, a surgery rotation, and then to a busy clinic where my late arrival was noticed with disapproval. After a three-hour session in an ice cold operating room, I took a break and limped by the cafeteria. The lunch special: fried chicken, mashed potatoes with gravy, creamed corn, and apple pie. Not on my diet, I thought. Then outside the residency office I noticed a sign on the bulletin board: "Radiology Case Studies, 6:30 p.m. to 9:30 p.m."

How could I even dream about eating right and getting back in shape with the way my day started, the cafeteria menu I just read, and the evening schedule I was facing? I was ready to give in again.

Later in the morning some unexpected inspiration came when a woman with a badly broken foot entered the clinic. Between the fighting children at her side and the note she asked me to write that would allow her to return to work early with crutches, the frustrations of my day lost their significance. Inspired by her tenacity, I started to rethink my defeatist attitude. It would have been so easy to blow off my good intentions, but her situation combined with the thought of another step backward and a longer road to fitness success was enough to change my mind.

So there I was with a food dilemma at lunch. I scavenged in the doctor's lounge, where I found some baby food with peaches and pears—not the perfect carbohydrate, but the price was right and the brand contained no added syrups or sugars. Finding some lean protein and vegetables was difficult, so I stripped the fried skin off of the chicken and placed the breast meat on top of some lettuce and tomatoes I grabbed from the hamburger station. Mid-afternoon, I found some plain tuna and ate it with some cottage cheese. Then at 5:00 p.m., I picked a few healthy jewels hidden among the usual grease-o-rama headliners at the cafeteria and placed them in a to-go container to avoid eating what I knew would be a calorie-fest at the lecture. Then I headed for the cardiology stress-testing floor where I was able to walk and jog on a treadmill for thirty minutes. After a few push-ups, sit-ups, and lunges, I hit the shower and ate my dinner during the radiology lecture that evening. Day accomplished, booby traps avoided!

That next morning I thought about all of the obstacles I had overcome and how it only took a little extra effort to stay the course. It would have been much easier to just give in to all the greasy, salty food choices that I was presented with throughout the day, and my busy schedule was the perfect excuse not to exercise. But thanks to a little inspiration, I didn't allow either to get in my way. Now, I was feeling my reward. I got out of bed feeling great the next day, and my muscles didn't ache. I guarantee that if I had eaten the usual cafeteria food I would have woken up feeling heavy and full. And if I hadn't stretched or walked on the treadmill, my muscles would still have been sore. And what had it taken? Just a decision, a choice—one that will become easier for you to make with your new Body of Knowledge.

Navigating the Obstacle Course

The key to winning the health and fitness game is planning a good defense and not to focus only on your eating and exercise offense. We all know about the wonderful advantages a healthy diet and exercise offer, but they won't help if you let obstacles confound you. It's not like we wake up one day and stop eating properly and quit exercising just because we are bored or unhappy with how great we look and feel. People drop out of diet and exercise programs because of the common intrusions of daily life. Muscles hurt. There is no time. It's too hard to find healthy food at work. Personal problems come up.

There is an endless supply of excuses. In fact, if it were just as easy to stick with a fitness program as it is to give in to excuses, we'd all be in great shape! But it's not. It all comes down to how each person deals with that convenient creature: the scapegoat. And since obstacles will always occur, your only recourse is to be able to recognize the most common pitfalls and know how to handle them.

Success is all about knowing the answers to questions like: What's going on with my body? Why do I feel like this? and How do I deal with it? So let's take a look at the obstacles standing in the way of our happy, healthiest selves.

Physical Obstacles

The most common physical difficulties—soreness, stiffness, burning, fatigue, cramping, and plateaus—are a direct result of, or a combination of, poor stretching habits, metabolic imbalances, temporary microscopic injury, tissue regeneration, or muscle recovery. Sounds like a lot to deal with, but you have already learned about most of these issues in Part 3. Other pitfalls such as slow progress or a slowing metabolism are also the result of simple biological phenomena. But there are simple ways to deal with these obstacles.

Soreness

You've probably already noticed that muscles tire and become sore approximately one to three days after exercise if you push it a little too hard. The body can typically handle slight changes in physical activity, but if you take on a weekend warrior attitude, look out! You could be uncomfortable for three to seven days or, worse, you'll be plagued with continual setbacks. If you stress and overexert unconditioned muscles, you will only lengthen the repair phase. That's why gradual staging is the best choice. A slow increase in activity over time will produce a tight feeling in your muscles during the repair stage, without excessive soreness. That's normal. In fact, most of my patients enjoy this feeling so much that they look forward to it and rarely push into the sore zone.

If you do go overboard and you find yourself quite sore in the days that follow:

- Stop exercising sore muscle groups for two, three, or ten days—whatever time it takes for that muscle group to recover and heal.
- Drink plenty of water—at least eight full glasses a day or use the suggestions in the BOK Ten Essential Tips for Weight Management. The water will help flush accumulated metabolite waste products out of your system.
- Apply ice to the affected area for twenty to thirty minutes, two to three times a day, for the first two to three days. Then start alternating ice and heat. Start with one minute hot and then immediately switch to cold for four minutes. Do this cycle four times (twenty minutes total) and always end with cold.
- Try using a heating pad before you exercise (not after) and do some slow stretching while you are resting until your soreness eases and you are left with only the tight feeling you usually feel after a good work out.

> IF YOU TAKE ON A WEEKEND WARRIOR ATTITUDE...YOU'LL BE PLAGUED WITH SETBACKS.

It is up to you to decide when to resume exercising the sore muscle group again, but I suggest that you wait until all discomfort has passed completely.

Stiffness

Stiffness is either a low level of soreness or something we rationalize as "getting older." It's a feeling of restriction that can involve any of the structures in our musculoskeletal system: muscles, tendons, or ligaments. It can feel like a thick rubber band that won't stretch very far. And it can affect one or several of these structures at the same time.

Maintaining your range of motion and limberness is one of the most important things you can do on a daily basis to maintain physical fitness. Morning, afternoon, evening, or any time you need a break, take your upper and lower body through a few stretches. It not only feels good, but can help you wake up in the morning, ease muscles after a workout, and reduce joint stiffness. As we get older a natural process called cross-linking, which we discussed in the chapter on BOK Switch Training, chemically bonds or fuses structures in our bodies when we are sedentary and decreases the elastic quality of our muscles, tendons, and joints. The only way to break or stop these bonds from forming is to eat a healthy diet, exercise regularly, and stretch.

> STRETCHING BEFORE OR AFTER EXERCISE … CARRIES NATURAL CHEMICALS TO MUSCLES … TO PREPARE THEM FOR ACTIVITY AND REPAIR THEM.

Warm up before any type of exercise, and cool down and stretch after. Stretching before or after exercise encourages blood flow, which brings heat to stiff and restricted body structures and makes them less prone to stress and strain. Blood flow also carries natural chemicals to muscles that are specifically designed to prepare them for activity and repair them after activity.

Fatigue and Burning

Burning during exercise is a part of muscle fatigue. The muscle has simply run out of gas—or metabolic energy. When pushed, your body may need more energy (remember ATP?). And there is also the build-up of acidic metabolites and lower levels of oxygen which also cause your muscles to burn.

Feeling tired or general fatigue can result from mental issues as well as physical, but improper nutrition, technique, and breathing are the main reasons muscles run out of steam. A low-carb diet or not eating sometime before exercise can also take the wind out of your sails. Remember, food is fuel. If you are experiencing any type of fatigue, review Parts 2 and 3 again and experiment with different food combinations, eating schedules, and exercise programs until you find what works best for you. Also, don't forget to watch your breathing. To this day I sometimes forget to breathe properly (especially when I am in a hurry), and what usually follows is a higher level of fatigue or lack of endurance.

Improper breathing can also lead to a burning sensation in your muscles while exercising as well, and can contribute to soreness afterward. As you know, proper breathing and blood flow can only supply your muscular demands to a certain extent, and then you'll begin to feel your limits. Your muscles may over-perform and require more oxygen than you can provide, or you may not deliver enough oxygen to them because of improper breathing techniques. Without enough oxygen to supply to your muscles during anaerobic exercise, lactic acid will begin to accumulate and you will experience a burning sensation. The good news is that stepping the workout down a notch, or switching to an aerobic exercise while focusing on proper breathing techniques, will reverse this process. That's because your body gets rid of lactic acid by converting it into carbon dioxide, which then escapes out of your lungs. The illustration on the next page shows the steps of this chemical process. You can go to the web site 🕮 to see the process with more detail.

> IMPROPER NUTRITION, TECHNIQUE, AND BREATHING ARE THE MAIN REASONS MUSCLES RUN OUT OF STEAM.

Pay attention to what is causing your fatigue and burning—then act on it. But as you become more conditioned, burning and fatigue will become less intense and easier to deal with. Even the type of exercise you choose (like BOK Switch Training) will minimize these effects. Just remember what you learned in Parts 2 and 3 about the importance of proper nutrition, breathing, repetitions, and technique.

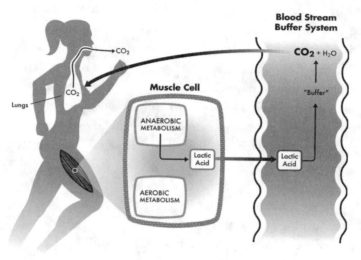

Cramping

I'm sure you have woken up in the middle of the night writhing in pain while you feel around for the ice pick that must be somewhere in the back of your calf. It's called a muscle cramp, and if you get one it is a sign of dehydration and an imbalance in the sodium, potassium, and pH (the acidity of blood) in your system. This in turn commingles with a lack of energy (ATP) and insufficient blood supply or oxygen delivery to the muscles. If a muscle does not have all the proper ingredients (especially enough ATP) to both contract *and* relax, then wham, you've got a cramp!

Cramps are most common in calf and foot muscles because they are farthest from the heart and lungs, which supply the muscles with the blood needed for them to function correctly. The best way to battle a calf muscle cramp is to get out of bed and slowly apply pressure downward on the ball of your foot while pulling your foot upward at the same time by contracting the muscles in the front of your leg. You can apply this technique with any muscle group that has a cramp. Go back to the chapter on BOK Switch Training in Part 3 and the web site to review the agonist-antagonist reflex for stretching and use it to your advantage. Remember that if you contract a muscle on the opposite side of a limb or joint, it will relax the muscle with the cramping force that is opposing it.

As for prevention, the best treatment uses the same stretching technique to stop the cramp, but you have to do it consistently. Forget pills and smelly sports creams. Instead stretch every night before you go to bed. If you are still having cramps, add another stretching session in the morning. Three sets per

> THE AGONIST-ANTAGONIST REFLEX ... WILL RELAX THE MUSCLE WITH THE CRAMPING FORCE.

leg and your cramps will be a thing of the past. Just don't forget that a proper balance of nutrition and hydration will also make a big difference.

Muscle Plateaus—What to Do When You're Stuck

As with anything in life, all good things must come to an end, or at least subside for a while. There you are, faithfully following your exercise regimen and joyfully experiencing continued success. And then one day everything comes to a screeching halt—despite your efforts. It's called "peaking" or reaching a muscle plateau, and it is one of the most discouraging obstacles for resistance-training enthusiasts.

Peaking is actually a good sign because it is announces that you have really made progress in your quest to improve your health and fitness. Peaking or plateaus are something you hear about in dieting but it is just as common, perhaps more common, in muscle development. People usually read this as either a sign that they have reached their maximum development potential or that they are not doing enough. Neither is correct. It is the body's way of saying, "Give me a break!" It is as if the body has a built-in safety mechanism protecting it from too much development too soon and too fast.

So, what should you do? Listen to your body and give it a rest. Because most people don't listen to their bodies, or don't have the knowledge, they see it as a sign to step up the work effort. Just the opposite is recommended.

A plateau is temporary. Remember, all the answers to health and fitness are locked up in our DNA somewhere; things like peaking happen for a reason. Muscle fibers can only grow so large and tendons, ligaments, and joints can only take so much stress before this protective reaction kicks in.

This is a good news, bad news, good news situation. Good news because now you know that a plateau is not a bad thing and your body just needs rest. Then a little bad news because you are going to have to rest and put your progress on hold. That means it will be necessary to lose some of the strength, size, and endurance that you worked so hard to achieve. But this brings on even better news. After a rest your body will be ready to return to its previous fitness level and have the ability to surpass it.

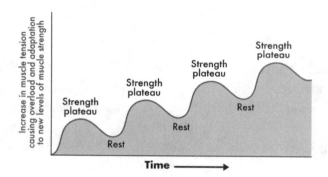

Most of us visualize muscle development as a steady climb, when in reality it is a cycle of peaks, plateaus, valleys, and more peaks. We just have to hold on to the knowledge that the results we desire will come, but we have to deal with some plateaus. You can make this newfound knowledge work for you by planning your "time off" around these plateaus. For example, I will make use of this knowledge every time I am either restricted by sedentary business commitments or on

> MUSCLE DEVELOPMENT... IS A CYCLE OF PEAKS, PLATEAUS, VALLEYS, AND MORE PEAKS.

my way to a vacation that is all about relaxation. I know it is healthy to back off my exercise a few times a year, so I simply plan accordingly. When I do get back into my workouts, I can either return gradually to my previous exercise level or step up the intensity and surpass it.

EXERCISE AND "FAT LAG TIME"

There may be a stage at the beginning or middle of your exercise or diet program when you feel like you aren't losing any fat. In fact, you might think you are actually gaining fat! Well, guess what? It's all true! Find out how "Fat Lag Time" works with eating and exercise to create this illusion on the web site.

How long the plateau will last differs for each individual and type of training. I have found that with resistance training a plateau can happen around the third to sixth month. As few as five and as many as fourteen days of rest is usually enough time to reset your body and return to your workout routine. Remember, as you read in Part 3, your muscles have a good memory. They know exactly where they left off and will be ready for their next challenge.

One way you can minimize muscle plateaus is to constantly change your workout. Different schedules may work better for some, but I recommend changing the type of exercise for each muscle group either every two weeks or alternating during the week. For example, you could change the type of exercises or switch from free weights to machines twice a month. You could also try to alternate your resistance training with Bikram yoga, Pilates, core training techniques, or other organized resistance training programs. Just a simple change in the types of exercise and areas of your muscles will remind them to continue building and keep you further from another plateau.

The Terrible Last Ten: Another Plateau?

Although the bathroom scale is never the absolute judge of your progress on the road to a new body, it can offer confirmation that you are making headway, especially during the early stages of fat loss.

With many people, particularly those who have a lot to lose, the first ten pounds seem to just fly right off. You just love that scale! Then it slows down—slow, slower, then even slower. And one day the scale just stops moving, refusing to budge no matter how hard you diet or how much extra time you spend at the gym. This is where a lot of diets end, often in disgust and disillusionment. So close, yet...

So why do so many people "get stuck" when they have only ten (or maybe more) pounds to lose? One reason is that long-term diet restrictions send a message to your body that it's headed for starvation, and consequently your metabolism slows. This is particularly true if you are restricting calories and not weight training. "Does dieting lower my metabolism?" is a question I get asked a lot when I lecture. The answer is yes (under the right circumstances). Find out how and why on the web site. As far as weight or "size" plateaus are concerned, trying too hard to eat too little can and will go against your goals. Serious diet restrictions make your body think its survival is threatened; as a result, it wants to store what energy it can.

Finally there is one more possibility that many of my patients overlook. Another reason for hitting a weight plateau just might be your body telling you that it is at the healthy weight it wants to be—as in, "Hey, get real. You look great!"

As I've said, the scale is never the absolute judge of your health or fitness. Remember that muscle weighs more than fat, so first evaluate exactly what you are trying to lose—pounds, inches, or poor health? Is your personal goal focused on a number, or is it about how you look and feel? If you are listening to the scale instead of the mirror or how you feel, or what your doctor says, then you are setting yourself up for failure.

If after evaluating how you look and feel, you really must to lose that last ten, then you need to reevaluate your eating and exercise program. It's likely, if you are at the "last ten" phase, you may not be as focused on your eating habits as you should be. Go back to the BOK Accelerated Fat Loss Meal Plan for a few weeks or temporarily apply some suggestions from the BOK – Quick Fix program in Part 4. This should help you get "unstuck."

If you are still not seeing the results you want, then take a look at the big picture, both past and present. In the beginning, all aspects of a diet and exercise regimen are usually quite focused, and your results are a direct reflection of your intensified efforts. As time passes your physical efforts may drop down a notch or two. Your current level of focus and enthusiasm may not be what it used to be—and that's okay. Just remember that there are always simple, logical reasons behind your successes and setbacks. Don't fall prey to assumptions that you are someone who has stubborn "fat genes" and are eternally damned with a "slow metabolism" or that you just don't have the ability to reach your goals.

There really is no secret to losing the terrible last ten, twenty, or more pounds. The reason is most likely one of the explanations above. Take a deep breath, reevaluate your goals and efforts, and you will see that this is just a simple plateau or an aggravation, not an obstacle. Sometimes standing still for a while or taking a few steps backward is what is necessary for you to start moving forward again.

Mental Obstacles

When I look back on one of the lower points of my life, I can picture myself sitting alone in front of the television and consuming a decadent meal loaded with fat, salt, and tons of sugar. I can also remember falling into bed like a load of bricks and sleeping far longer than normal. I didn't feel rested when I woke up, I had no desire whatsoever to exercise nor was I feeling good about myself in general.

I am sure most of you know exactly what I am talking about. Of all the obstacles to good health and fitness, the mental ones are the hardest to overcome. Let's examine what they are and why they're a problem, and what we can do to keep our mental commitment to a healthy life on track.

Sweet Demise: Carbs, Fatigue, and the Mood Blues

I can think of no great saboteur to a healthy eating plan than a sugar binge. Sugar, a simple carbohydrate, is the reason carbohydrates have gained a reputation as a "bad for you" food and was the catalyst for the recent onslaught of low-carb products. But remember what we've learned: you can't lump all carbs together or eliminate an entire fuel group from your healthy diet.

Complex carbohydrates, like vegetables and whole grains, are actually some of the best foods Mother Nature has to offer. Like fruits, they also contain simple carbs, but in a natural, time-released form. It is the simple, processed carbs, such as sugar, white flour, and other refined foods, that give carbs a bad rap. But when it comes to thwarting good eating intentions, sugar, well, takes the cake. No wonder desserts spelled backward is stressed!

You've already learned in Part 2 how an influx of simple carbs causes the pancreas to release too much insulin and sends your blood sugar on a reckless swing of highs and lows, creating a craving for sweets followed by an energy slump followed by another craving for more sweets.

And the negative effects of carbohydrate abuse go beyond the physical; they can cause mental turmoil as well. Chronic consumption of simple carbohydrates—ice cream, candy, cookies, and other sugary sweets—has been linked to mood swings, chronic mental fatigue, anxiety, and even depression. More proof that food is, in essence, a drug. How sugar can produce such dramatic psychological changes is still being investigated, but researchers are finding more evidence that it may be a chicken-or-egg situation. Sugar abuse can cause a negative state of mind which can then cause a sugar binge. Unfortunately, it is a vicious cycle of hunger, sugar cravings, eating, and crashing. It is an insidious cycle of highs and lows that is tough to break.

Give in to a sugar craving too often for too long and you will settle into a rut of fatigue that will have you on the couch instead of in the gym. And then you'll be angry with yourself. In your disgusted state of mind, you may seek refuge in the cookie jar.

CAN POOR EATING HABITS CREATE DEPRESSION?

According to the American Psychiatric Association, many people tend to eat voraciously during their lowest point of depression, which usually coincides with their lowest blood sugar levels. That leads me to the question: can poor eating habits create depression, even for those who are not overweight? I believe that a poor diet can and does affect behavior in certain situations. And there is plenty of research involved with this vicious cycle of depression and overeating.

The truth of the matter is that everyone enjoys a little overindulgence from time to time. Just use your sensible discipline skills and learn to allow an occasional overindulgence—that is, unplanned and spontaneous when life offers it. But if overeating becomes more frequent (bingeing is defined as overeating, on average, at least two days a week for six months) and gives you a "let-down" feeling, then it is affecting you mentally. Step back, take a look at the big picture, and make an effort to straighten things out by focusing on healthy habits first. If things don't turn around or seem like they are out of control it is best get a jump on this and consult a professional counselor. Sometimes just a little early intervention can not only prevent a large setback but can also reverse a more difficult situation more rapidly and with less stress. Don't jump to conclusion yet, though. We will go over the signs and symptoms for this and other common dysfunctions and disorders more in Surviving the Cerebral Jungle. And don't forget that the knowledge you already have gives you a big advantage over the average person. A healthy diet and exercise plan is a critical part of all professional mental health treatment programs.

You can also use your eating knowledge tools to prepare for events that trigger your problems. Whether you are facing a critical business meeting or anticipating an important social event, knowing how different foods affect your body and mind will allow you to plan for any situation. If your plans change, so can your eating habits. Manage your life before life manages you. And that includes managing your time.

Managing Time
"I didn't have time."

Everyone has used time as an excuse for not doing something important, and most people will continue to do so. It's true, time is a convenient excuse because there are only twenty-four hours in a day. We can't create more time or change it—or can we?

I try to make time work for me as much as possible, and smart time management is the starting point. Think of time management as a recipe for success with the key ingredients consisting of your priorities. Priorities change as time marches on. Major time commitments, such as time with family and friends, vary only slightly through the years. Work, exercise, and diet priorities, however, can change daily.

Some of you may have the gift of automatic prioritization, allowing you to manage your day or your work without stress or effort. Yours truly, on the other hand, needs to think things through first. If it's jotting down your weekly schedule every Sunday night or going over your day during your morning coffee, it's worth every second. With the advent of hand held devices, cell phones and software programs like Microsoft Outlook, you can make your time spent on management more efficient because your information is easy to access and automatic reminders take care of your occasional forgetfulness. Time management is all about organization, and both are directly dependent on how you set your priorities. And maintaining your overall health should always be one of your top priorities. If it's not, you will have a very difficult time with the rest of your priorities.

MAKE A TO-DO LIST

If you are like most twenty-first century Americans, you attempt to keep pace with the speed of daily life by keeping a to-do list. I know I do, and I rarely go home at night without crossing off the top five items. A few times a week one of my top three priorities is a single word: exercise. My adage is simple: just do *something*. Is exercise on your to-do list? I don't have to remind myself to eat well every day because it is what I do naturally (after twenty years of trial and error). But if there is something coming up on a certain day that will interfere with my healthy eating regimen, then eating healthily goes to the top of my list. Do I need to take my lunch to work tomorrow because the cafeteria menu doesn't suit me? Do I need to stop at the market on the way home? Do I need to find or recommend a restaurant that serves the kind of food I want? If so, they go right to the top of my to-do list. Always put your health and fitness needs at the top of your to-do list and everything else will fall into place.

The key to time management is efficiency—fine-tuning your life. One of the most inefficient things I find in life is commuting. I think we forget how important geography is to time management. But until we can transport ourselves from place to place like they do on Star Trek, traveling may be one of the most time-consuming things in our lives.

You have probably developed some of your own time-saving travel habits, but just for fun, let's look at a few of my favorite time savers for diet and exercise.

1. Work out at home, the office, or choose a gym that has several locations locally or nationally. This will allow you to squeeze exercise in when your time is limited, such as during your lunch hour, between errands, or when you travel.

2. Lift weights only on the days when daily travel takes you by the health club or other workout destination. A trip home between work and workout could double your travel time or invite a temptation to stay home and skip the gym.

3. Always keep a bag with a change of clothes in your car or at work so you are prepared for an unexpected stretch of free time when you could exercise.

4. Have several types of exercise equipment at home (barbell, dumbbells, Swiss ball, bike, roller blades, jump rope, cushioned mat, etc.) to maintain variety and so you have the mobility to adapt to location and weather changes.

5. Change into your workout clothes at work. It will keep you from making excuses on your way to the gym.

> THE KEY TO TIME MANAGEMENT IS EFFICIENCY.

6. Pack healthy snacks the night before and leave a reminder on your computer, by your briefcase, wallet, purse, or handbag so you remember to take your snack in the morning. Even better, if you have a place to store them, bring a collection of healthy snacks to the office once a week so that they are always on hand.

7. Prepare a larger quantity of healthy food once or twice during the week so you don't have to do it daily. Cook in double batches and seal up the rest in containers or zip-lock bags—cook once, eat twice!

8. Consider taking classes at your gym (body sculpting, spinning, cross-training, swimming, etc.) once or twice a week. Try to think of the classes as appointments that you can't miss. They will keep your time at the gym limited, and you will usually get a well-rounded workout with motivation from the instructor.

9. Prepare a meal list before you go shopping for the week. You'll spend less time at the grocery store and less time each day figuring out what you're going to eat.

Many of these steps may seem obvious, but if you follow them consistently you'll see the benefits.

Paper or Plastic—How Do You Organize?

More and more lately, it seems as if I lose track of my priorities or simply forget important tasks. I've not only found the television remote control in my refrigerator in the morning, but I've watched my frozen yogurt melting in the shopping cart because I spent too much time in the store without a list and then forgot where I parked the car. We just don't function well when we have too many things on our minds, and organizing our tasks can help tremendously.

Let's face it, the world has become a very busy place, and organization is our only salvation. This is especially true when it comes to information management. What's your favorite form of record keeping? Is it making notes in a spiral notebook or your diary? Maybe you prefer to click away on the plastic keys of your personal computer or convenient hand-held device. If I don't write myself reminders and keep detailed records, important tasks go by the wayside and chaos takes over. The same holds true for your diet and exercise goals.

In your quest for a healthy body, you will encounter both positive and negative reactions to certain exercises and eating behaviors. Write them down! If you wake up one day feeling absolutely great, take a look at what you ate and what exercises you did a day or two before to find out what contributed to the energy you have today. On the other hand, if you find yourself struggling in the gym or feel tired during the day, important information might be in your BOK Journal that will give you clues to the cause (Go to the web site ⌨ to print as many journal pages as you need). One day, halfway through a workout, I couldn't believe how good I felt and how much energy I had. After some thought, I determined that it was the food combination I ate in the car thirty minutes before I arrived at the gym. I looked it up in my journal so I could try it again.

The more information you document, the better. Note the type and variety of exercises you do, what you eat, the time of day you exercise, what you eat before and after exercise, and any new exercise technique or food you try.

Most importantly, document how you feel, including both your mental and physical energy levels. If you can't commit to daily record-keeping, at least take notes on the instances when you have extremely good or bad experiences.

A journal or personal database is an important tool for your Body of Knowledge program and long-term success. The thought of documenting your findings may seem like overdoing it at first, but in time it will prove to be invaluable. Once you have truly reflected on your daily, weekly, or monthly results, you will be able to reach your goals faster and easier, and have better odds of maintaining those results.

Stop-Loss Priorities

Our functional "extra time" is what's left of our daily twenty-four hours after sleep and work. How you use this time is up to you, and it's all about priorities. Again, I urge you to put your health at the top of the priority list and give it the time it deserves.

I know from experience that people can get overwhelmed if they feel they are faced with too many responsibilities that require a high level of time and effort. They will end up doing nothing. When faced with this situation, your best option is to pick the top one or two priorities that are both time and result effective—I call these stop-loss priorities.

These are the most important items that not only produce better overall results, but they are usually the ones that provide the best bang for your buck or need to be execut-

> SKIPPING KEY STOP-LOSS PRIORITIES WILL SET YOU BACK IN YOUR GOALS.

ed before other important tasks can be performed at all. To get right to the point, skipping key stop-loss priorities will set you back the farthest and fastest. It may be a quick visit to the grocery store to stock up on healthy food for work or critical exercises in your fundamental resistance training program—make these stop-loss priorities happen.

If you only have time for a few of these in a particular week, there is one stop-loss priority that will maximize your time and minimize any setbacks. What I want you to do is simply take a few minutes each evening and make both time management and time efficiency a high stop-loss priority. This will continue to flush out the critical tasks for the next day, week, or month.

Don't cheat yourself out of good health. Don't compromise the one thing that will make you happier and healthier. Most importantly, making more time for *your* health and well-being will also benefit your family and friends—don't cheat them too.

Surviving the Cerebral Jungle

Have you ever felt out of control, like your body does what it wants even though your mind intends otherwise? Do you ever get a sudden and overwhelming feeling of stress, excitement, or unhappiness and crave comfort food?

So what sets off these cravings? How do our emotions get involved in the first place? When we're down, we want comfort, and many times food fills that void—anything that tastes good and makes us "feel better." When we're feeling high we celebrate with alcoholic beverages, extravagant feasts, and decadent desserts. Stress can make us robotically empty a can of chips without taking notice. Food and emotion just go hand in hand in our culture.

For people with more serious eating problems, food is actually a bad side effect to their emotional situations. It becomes the drug of choice for suppressing (or escaping) or enhancing the emotional experience at hand. And while most of us would simply say that our eating habits are not as healthy as we would like, there are those who cannot distinguish an unhealthy eating habit from the unhealthy emotional cycle that is linked to it. Just in the last few decades, abnormal eating habits or eating disorders have received more attention in mainstream media and medicine.

Eating disorders are now out in the open, receiving the attention necessary to find management techniques and cures. They have become easier to recognize and have better treatment protocols. And the common eating disorders, such as bulimia and anorexia, do not represent the entire spectrum of unhealthy relationships with food.

There are other problems that fall between normal, healthy eating habits and eating disorders. I call these problems dysfunctional eating habits. Sub-classifications probably exist, but I believe that all of you reading this book will see at least a little of yourself in this general classification.

Emotions and Food: The Tie That Unravels

Remember Tracy? She was the classic loser and gainer who didn't reach permanent success until she was able to face the personal issues that drove her to the refrigerator in the first place. It took courage and hard work, but her decision to change was the key. Change is a scary thing. Many of us react to change with fear, anger, or resistance—a typical response in modern society. Giving up comfortable habits or traditions is hard, but being unhealthy and unhappy is much harder. Tracy would have been among the 90 to 95 percent attrition rate—dieters who fail to maintain their weight loss—if she had not finally recognized her emotional link to food.

If you want to succeed as Tracy did and make your new, healthy lifestyle your permanent lifestyle, then finding the emotional triggers that contribute to your struggles with health and fitness is the first critical step. Half of the problem is solved by adhering to the eating and exercise suggestions you have already read. The other half is having a plan to "stick with it" and maintain your progress when unhealthy influences threaten your healthy changes. It is so important to have a game plan for both of these challenges that I recommend that you do not begin your journey until you prepare for these inevitable setbacks and obstacles. It's a simple formula. First determine what you need to do and then determine how you are going to keep doing it.

Today the behavior modification portion of weight management is becoming a standard part of all programs. Think of your plan as an extended warranty on your new machine. A personal investment now will ensure a better future and minimize your chances of returning to old habits. In fact, the successful "re-entry" programs (which prevent relapsing or address resurfacing issues) are making a healthy diet and exercise plan mandatory for other unhealthy habits, such as drug addiction and alcoholism. Simply put, they work.

Break the Addiction

As you now know, the body is designed to operate optimally on healthy fuel mixtures of protein, fats, and carbohydrates, but unfortunately, it can still operate on an unhealthy diet. That's the problem. This wonderful machine that carries us through life is very resourceful and incredibly resilient. Not only can we manufacture fat from carbohydrates and burn protein when needed, we can still manage to motor on some of the most unhealthy and non-nutritious foods imaginable.

Many people with extremely poor eating habits, obese or otherwise, will tell you that they physically and mentally "feel okay." Their machines have adjusted to their unhealthy lifestyles and will continue fighting to keep functioning normally. In fact, I had one 400-pound patient tell me that he didn't mind the few inconveniences his size caused. But, as you can surmise, it is just a matter of time before overabundance takes over and starts to break the machine down. We have been bombarded for years with scientific proof linking poor eating habits to health problems.

So, why do some people continue to eat so poorly?

Because for some food is an addiction as wicked as any addiction to illegal drugs. In many ways, it is worse because this "drug" is in endless, legal supply.

DID YOU KNOW THAT OUR BODIES MAKE DRUGS? FIND OUT MORE ON THE WEB SITE. 📖

Consider this: We introduce children to sugar practically the minute they go on solid food. They lose out on the nutrients and energy they would get from the foods they should be eating—complex carbs in fruits and vegetables (with natural vitamins and minerals), the stuff the body was designed to run on. The result is a no-win energy balance that favors storing calories instead of burning them. Even worse, some children have sensitivities or don't have the proper machinery to process these simple carbohydrates and could be headed for serious health problems, such as hypoglycemia or diabetes.

A direct injection of pure sugar also upsets the natural balance of their brains' reward mechanisms, creating a dependency and a substance abuse syndrome as strong as any drug addiction. Sugar is just like alcohol, cigarettes, coffee, marijuana, or cocaine—concentrated forms of naturally occurring plant products that are chemically intensified and altered for reasons that have nothing to do with promoting good health.

Simple Carbohydrates: Food Drug of Choice

Most unprocessed and even processed carbohydrates started life with good intentions. The common white sugar we are most familiar with is processed from sugar cane or sugar beets, two plants found in nature. Chemically, these plants are mainly composed of complex carbohydrates and natural sugars.

But at some point in time, man got the idea that heating and stripping these plants of their natural fiber, water, vitamins, and minerals would create a product that would taste better and have a longer shelf-life in the grocery store. Refined sugar was born, the chemically altered simple carbohydrate that is in almost every processed food we eat. It is recognized and burned as fuel and it is also very addictive.

The addiction to sugar begins with the stimulation it gives your taste buds. This intensified carbohydrate signal then travels to other parts of your brain, including the brain stem, where your strongest and most primitive instincts reside—pleasure and survival. Even though there is biochemical mayhem going on in your body after a large dose of the sweet stuff, the survival message your primitive brain stem receives is "Sugar good. Me no starve."

Refined sugar not only bypasses the natural carbohydrate breakdown process which regulates how it is burned or stored but it also intensifies a natural "reward cycle" that is part of your most primal brain. When this area in your brain stem is stimulated by normal amounts of non-processed carbs, there is a positive mental response that releases mood enhancers like serotonin and reinforces your choice to eat carbohydrates—a healthy chemical reward. Yes, even non-processed complex carbs can act like a drug, but they evoke a lower reward stimulus that goes unnoticed when you eat smaller, healthy portions.

With refined sugar and other processed carbs, the intensified reward stimulus not only creates a "high" that you would like to revisit but also tells your survival instincts that this is a really good way to stay alive! In short, your body will never tell you to turn extra calories away because of the joy they bring to your taste buds and brain stem.

Sugar Withdrawals

Sugar addiction is a tough cycle to break because…it's everywhere! And when you decide to kick the habit, there is another roadblock, one that also supports and maintains the addiction cycle—withdrawals.

As with drugs, kicking the sugar habit and other comfort foods means going through withdrawals. Initially your body will fight against giving up the physical and mental feelings that sugar produces. The physical withdrawal symptoms begin and then the mental cravings follow. Most of our natural cravings are fine, but we have all seen or experienced the intense power of a dessert, candy, or bread craving. Not only do we sometimes close our eyes and say "mmm" while devouring something sweet, but the whole decadent act is preceded by an inner cry of "I gotta have it!" So next time you see a child throwing a tantrum at a grocery store candy display, hopefully the usual irritation will be replaced with pity for their cravings and withdrawals.

So how do you break the cycle? The first step is to understand that it isn't easy. But if you resist temptation and begin to eat properly—in quantity and quality—the stressful feelings of the withdrawal will pass with time, and a healthy, calm feeling will take over. And, as long as you continue these healthy eating habits, the feeling of good health will take hold permanently.

Getting there requires you to put your newfound knowledge into action. You don't have to just tough it out though. Slowly remove these "drugs" from your diet and minimize the dose when you do fall prey to their cravings. Of course, like any addictive drug, the best solution is to completely get it out of your life. But that is hardly a reality with the abundance of available processed carbohydrates.

> **LEARN ABOUT THE PAST AND FUTURE OF WEIGHT-LOSS MEDICATION ON THE WEB SITE.** **ARE THERE SMARTER DRUGS?**

Carbohydrates, good and not so good, remain members of one of our three fuel sources, so "no carbs" is not the answer either—just pay attention to moderation and healthy combinations of carbohydrates for weight management and wellness. One successful technique for handling a sugar craving is to combine sweets with unprocessed carbohydrates or fiber. It will help minimize the physical and mental effects. A small amount of fat or protein added to a simple carb is also better than eating it alone. The combinations will minimize both the insulin response and infamous "sugar crash" that makes you want more. Experiment and find out what works best for you.

Discovering the source of your cravings is the next step. Once you know what triggers an unhealthy craving and the effect it has on your mind and body, you can start to remove its power over you. And during this process, you will gradually make smarter choices without much thought or effort. Before long, choices will become instinct.

Again, it all comes down to knowledge—the best rehab program in town.

Dysfunctional Eating Habits

So what are dysfunctional eating habits, and how do they come about?

They come in all forms but usually have harmless titles like routines, and family traditions, passed down without much thought from generation-to-generation like jewelry or a fruitcake recipe. Although serious eating disorders are more damaging to our overall health, dysfunctional eating habits are not to be taken lightly and also need to be addressed in order to make progress toward a healthy lifestyle. Often, just recognizing them or identifying their influence will halt any setbacks they have caused in the past. Other times it may take a little more perseverance and practice or maybe some counseling to figure out where they came from or what exactly is dysfunctional.

Food, Family, and the "Double Bind"

One of the most common dysfunctional eating habits is what I call the "finish everything on your plate" syndrome. In practically every family, children are coaxed to finish the food they are given, whether they are hungry or not. Some families use bribes or extortion, such as "…or you can't watch TV" and worse, "…or you can't have dessert." It's a habit born of good intention, initiated by caring parents concerned about finicky eaters. What many parents don't realize is that many times their children can't finish their food because instinctively they are already full and know it's time to stop eating. What's even more disheartening is the guilt that is used to push the demand along. "There are starving children in…" Some persistent parents will make children sit in exile alone at the dinner table with threats of extra chores or something worse. Then when they finally do finish their food, the uncomfortable, stuffed feeling it produces is rewarded with acceptance, praise, or even a hug. And it can produce one of the most common psychological cycles of love association children can develop, one that can follow them throughout their adult lives:

Full = Love

This and other examples that follow fall under the umbrella of what psychiatric experts call the double bind. A double bind is a "no way out" situation that places a person in a quagmire comprised of stress, guilt, shame, and fear. In the scenario I just described, the parents are creating the double bind by repeatedly making a demand supported by threats that conflict with the child's natural instincts and logical assumption (that it's time to stop eating). But this is only one of the essential elements of a double bind situation. Of course, the parents are just passing on a tradition from their own upbringing and are doing it out of love. On the surface it seems admirable—parents ensuring their children's good health by making sure that they finish all of their food. What it really does is place children in a mental tug of war between what they feel is right and wrong. Their instincts are telling them that they are full, but mom or dad is telling them that this is not right. The matter is further complicated with other double bind elements like guilt (starving children in…) or even extortion-fear (no television, no dessert). The result is confusion and a desire for the uncomfortable situation to go away. It can also cause a hatred for otherwise healthy foods, causing kids to gorge on snack foods when away from home.

After the child is "broken" and these after-dinner disputes fade away, the pattern becomes an accepted way of life. Finishing a large plate of food avoids family stress and evokes admiration. That's when the other destructive eating cycle starts. Both physically and mentally

A DOUBLE BIND IS A "NO WAY OUT" SITUATION… COMPRISED OF STRESS, GUILT, SHAME AND FEAR.

it will always feel good to eat everything on the plate when eating smaller portions, larger portions, or all you can eat buffets with family, friends, or alone.

WARNING SIGNS OF UNHEALTHY EATING PATTERNS

Do the following statements sound familiar?

- Every time I eat, I worry I am making myself fat.
- Sometimes, I won't eat when I am hungry.
- Sometimes, I eat so much I feel sick.
- I eat even when I am not hungry, like when I'm bored.
- I often feel guilty about what I eat.
- When I overeat, I exercise a lot to make up for the extra calories.
- Everyone tells me I am thin, but I know I need to lose weight.

Punishment and Reward

"Finish everything on your plate" is not the only double bind game in town, though. Other combinations of food and punishment can have stronger effects. Furthermore, they are not only damaging to a child's overall physical and mental health, but certain double bind situations are linked to more serious schizophrenic symptoms. Similar damage is done when parents use food as reward. Children will connect the love, affection, and praise from a parent with the chemical reward the brain receives from the food. And then some parents take it to the next level: using the reward becomes a tool of extortion. "No ice cream if you're bad" sends a the stronger signal of fear to a child that he or she will not be loved and accepted, because love and acceptance is associated with food. The cycle is reinforced because ice cream (or any food) becomes a drug that stimulates the reward center in the brain. The child, and eventually when they are an adult, uses the food as a reward, as a down payment for future tasks when he or she is sick, or for comfort.

The worst situation of all is the practice of taking food away as punishment. It leaves a child feeling scared, unaccepted, unloved, and above all, unnourished. Now the instinct of survival is threatened, which evokes the strongest emotions and causes a heightened level of fear. The final outcome is an extremely damaging and powerful cycle and an unhealthy association between food and self-image.

Break the cycle. Replace food with communication. Talk with your children about the problem in question and simply make them accountable for their actions, such as paying for a vandalized object by working after school or more study time and less television when grades drop. There are so many other healthy options for rewarding your family that remove the food association and addiction. Replace the trip to the ice cream shop with one to the arts and crafts store. Instead of the dessert in front of the television, create some family memories and play an interactive board game. Not only will you maintain your intimacy and closer bonds with your family, but your children will be more likely to excel in school and other extracurricular activities.

> THE WORST SITUATION OF ALL IS ... TAKING FOOD AWAY AS PUNISHMENT..

And for us adults with or without children at home, keep in mind that these childhood examples are all a part of our lives, too. They resonate in our minds and bodies, often without our awareness. Those of you who have children may rationalize dysfunctional eating habits by reliving your past through them or joining in the cycle blindly. But even when there is no one around, too often the desire to feel loved, safe, and happy ends up with a trip to the pantry.

PRESSURES AWAY FROM HOME

Eating rituals that lead to poor health occur away from home as well. Desire for popularity and acceptance and easy access to unhealthy foods contribute to the problem.

Children share chips, candy, ice cream, fast food, and other unhealthy snacks as a way of trying to fit in with their peers and identify with the slogans and images from advertisements. Then the baton is passed on to adulthood and another round of unhealthy habits appears. In most workplaces, there are candy jars in reception areas, doughnuts brought in for morning meetings, power lunches, power dinners, happy hours, and after-work socials. There is no shortage of food or alcohol (and its disinhibition). Many people feel that if they try to avoid these events it would be detrimental to their careers. Sometimes saying "no" is difficult, but no amount of acceptance is worth your good health.

Speed Eating

Speed eating is another dysfunctional habit that contributes to unhealthy eating patterns. As you've learned, it takes twenty minutes for the satiety center in the brain to recognize what you've eaten. Speed eaters can inhale an awful lot of calories in twenty minutes.

Speed eating is learned at an early age when the family hurries to finish breakfast so that everyone can rush off to school or work and continues at dinner when everyone hurries to finish in order to rush off to evening events or to plop in front of the television. In our minds, eating quickly avoids stress, offers success, and sends a greater than normal signal of satisfaction to the brain—another cycle that's tough to stop. Think like many of our European neighbors and savor your time, your family, your friends, and your food at the dinner table. Slow down, take breaks, and replace the shoveling with conversation.

Dysfunctional eating habits are hard to avoid. They are like little traps we fall into if we don't watch where we are going. And combined with a sedentary lifestyle, they contribute to the growing problem of obesity. I encourage you to start by recognizing the habits that we have reviewed—knowing you have a bad habit is the first step to correcting it. Don't let a dysfunctional eating habit grow into an eating disorder.

HOLIDAYS: TRICKS OR TREATS?

Americans love to celebrate and in typical American style—we figure the bigger the better. Thanksgiving takes the cake...or the pumpkin pie. One of my most vivid childhood memories is the circus of events that took place in my home leading up to the feast. Days of shopping, chopping, slicing, cooking, baking, linen washing, and silver polishing led up to the hour or so it took to polish off the meal. At the Moore house, there was even an unspoken competition to see who could go beyond a third helping. And then, of course, the desserts would arrive, which was like viewing a 40-carat blue diamond—with lots of oohs and aahs. Finally we celebrated by lumbering to the couches where another tradition would unfold: writhing in pain from being overstuffed, and admonishments for eating too much!

This may be only a once or twice a year phenomenon for your family too, but there are families that adopt a Thanksgiving-like attitude to family meals on a frequent, even daily, basis. In some families, it is a ritual. And when it starts in childhood, it may become a way of life that is tough to correct.

Eating Disorders

The dysfunctional eating habits I have described don't have their own specific scientific classifications, self-help groups, or certified medical treatment programs, but the more serious eating disorders do and for good reason. In the past, these disorders were viewed as mental diseases. Relatives or friends would quietly smuggle the afflicted person to an institution or rehabilitation program for help.

The diagnosis and treatment of eating disorders have come a long way and are now more commonly recognized and treated in mainstream medicine. Research has even found a link between these disorders and other health problems, such as heart disease, diabetes, high blood pressure, cystic fibrosis, inflammatory bowel disease, Crohn's disease, thyroid problems, and various forms of cancer.

It is promising that eating disorders have been receiving more attention in America and other countries lately. Although most of you will not have all of the symptoms and signs of any particular eating disorder, at least be able to recognize them to protect yourself from heading down that path. And if you do recognize the signs or symptoms in your own behavior and habits, you will be informed enough to seek the proper advice or treatment.

There are many varieties of eating disorders, but most are related in some way to two primary disorders: anorexia nervosa (characterized by the absence or near absence of eating) and bulimia nervosa (characterized by an eat-and-purge cycle). The various forms of these conditions are classified according to signs, symptoms, diagnoses, and compliancy during diagnosis and treatment.

If you want to see more information about psychological criteria for some of the most common eating disorders, go to the web site [📖], but please *do not try to diagnose yourself.*

You may recognize some of the elements in your own behavior. If you believe that you may have an eating disorder, it is critical that you speak to a doctor right away. An eating disorder is not easy to diagnose or cure, and you can't do it on your own.

> THE DIAGNOSIS AND TREATMENT OF EATING DISORDERS ARE NOW... RECOGNIZED AND TREATED IN MAINSTREAM MEDICINE.

Fear, Anger, Shame, and Guilt

Four of the primary emotions that fuel the eating disorder fires are fear, anger, shame, and guilt. These emotions in all their different degrees begin and maintain the cycle that leads to an unhealthy relationship with food. Eating disorders are like other physical illnesses, but unlike other more common health problems, there aren't simple pills, operations, or rehabilitation equipment to cure them.

Treatment of eating disorders is not all about food, though; food is not the focal point of the problem. In fact, there are usually several problems associated with an eating disorder, and they vary greatly from individual to individual. Food may fuel the vehicle that takes a person to his or her eating disorder destination, but the addictive cycles that develop is what keeps them there. Treatment requires going to the source of the problems—ourselves—and then finding the unhealthy connections that are outside of ourselves. My mother uses the adage "It takes two to tango," and it couldn't be more appropriate here.

People with eating disorders are frequently surrounded by others who have helped them develop or continue to support their problems with food. For the person with the disorder, it is difficult to understand how others contributed to a problem that they only connect to food until they take a good look at a critical part of childhood development.

Because the problem is central to the family unit and families tend to stick together, there is no escape. The child with the developing eating disorder has nowhere to go and only one choice: to accept the cycle and all those who are involved. And to compound the problem, a child's view of the world from a self-centered perspective can create some unhealthy conclusions. They feel that their behaviors are related to all emotions within the family—that even the discomfort and stress that develops is their fault. This is no one's fault and is not something that can be "fixed." As babies develop into young children, they perceive themselves as the origin for everything that they see and do. In fact, they do not begin to fully recognize others separate from their world and understand their influence on their lives until kindergarten or grammar school.

THE EVOLUTION OF FEAR, ANGER, SHAME, AND GUILT

During the first few years of life, we recognize little outside of our basic needs for survival and those who provide for those needs. Initially we see all things in our world as loving and nurturing. Take that outlook and combine it with the fact that almost every action we take at this early age is a natural action. If whatever we do is met with a positive response, it creates a cycle of love, trust, and acceptance. This cycle is altered when something is labeled as "bad" (like finger painting on the wall). Eventually we learn that certain "bad" behaviors do not deliver the nurturing responses we seek. And in some cases the new bewildered feeling that results from this disapproval is ramped up to discomfort or pain with an added negative reinforcement (such as a time-out or a spanking).

We quickly learn to stay away from a new situation that does not feel good or leads to negative consequences with a little help from the emotion called fear. But what if something that is a natural instinct that feels good to a child is labeled as "bad"? Ta da! The child is introduced to the feelings of shame and guilt. Shame is awakened when the child performs the "bad" act again and suffers punishment or disapproval as a result. Guilt often follows once the shame associated with a behavior has passed, or when the child performs the bad act again, with or without being caught. Anger is introduced directly by example (angry parents or guardians) and indirectly by persistent double bind situations that frustrate the child to the breaking point. To make matters worse, children are fast learners, and they learn to use fear, anger, shame, and guilt in dealing with their parents or guardians, which creates a vicious cycle—unless there is some sort of intervention.

Children are incredibly resilient and tenacious, though, so rather than give up, they look for a solution. They try to fix the problem, but learn that they cannot fix anyone else. Most kids then determine that the only way to get rid of the discomfort or painful feelings is to keep them under control. And since young children conclude that they are the source of their problems, they find ways to control aspects of their own lives.

There are many ways of creating a sense of control in one's life, but eating disorders are one of the most common. In reality, control over the body may be a false sense of control, but it does not seem that way to the person with this problem. Eating less or more helps a person with an eating disorder control uncomfortable and painful feelings with that wonderful, legal drug: food. Food is the vital tool that enables adults and children to control their body, their world, their daily discomforts, and the painful situations that seem focused on them. This need for control can lead to the two main eating disorder classifications, anorexia and bulimia. As the following flow chart indicates, the situation becomes a cycle of addiction. Addiction and control go hand in hand. And the drug (food in this case) is <u>not</u> the cause, just a physical link in this emotional cycle.

As you can see, an addiction cycle is very complex. And when you are in such a cycle, there is no room for rational analysis on your behalf. The cycle becomes a natural reaction or reflex that governs your actions—so natural that you (and possibly many of the people in your life) do not recognize it as abnormal.

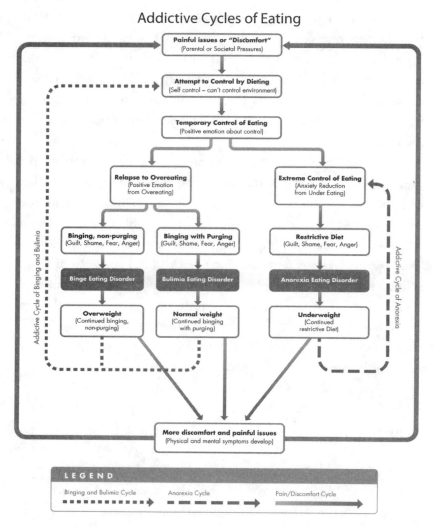

Addictive Cycles of Eating

Action and Reaction

Fear, anger, shame, and guilt are simply emotional *reactions*. But it is the *actions* that cause these reactions that are central to treating an eating disorder. One of the most common actions at the root of eating disorders is *abuse*, whether mild or severe. It is estimated that 80 percent of people with an eating disorder have experienced some sort of abuse as a child and/or as an adult. All forms of abuse—emotional, verbal, physical, or sexual—can cause enough pain and discomfort to trigger these disorders. Believe it or not, intense emotional or verbal abuse can create the same problems that physical or sexual abuse provoke.

Sadly, children will blame themselves for the abuse. Sometimes they feel responsible even if abuse is directed at someone else in a family. The fact that they cannot leave the family setting perpetuates the problem and its four-pronged reactions. Abuse creates its own cycle, too. Sometimes, children come to view abusive behavior as a sign of love and caring. Although one could imagine that verbal abuse could be accepted as an intense level of concern and caring, it seems odd to think that sexual abuse could be viewed as a loving act. Love and comfort is what all children seek and expect from their families, and they will find that love in any type of attention they get. Adult abusers have most definitely had some level of abuse in their own upbringings. Even if they can acknowledge the damage it caused in their lives, they somehow continue to commit the same abuse or other unpleasant situations they experienced, passing it down to the next generation.

Hard to believe, but simple disapproval of a child's emotions can also be damaging. One example is a parent telling a child to stop crying. The child reads the command as a signal that the parent does not care what he or she is crying about, or worse, that the pain or emotion causing the crying is his or her fault, hence the parent's angry reaction. The punishment that sometimes follows when the child does not stop crying is another common and potent double bind situation. Even ignoring children who are asking for attention sends a similar message of disapproval.

In the end, it is a child's feelings in relationship to what he or she sees and encounters that regulate reactions and actions as he or she matures. They define a child's perception of comfort and love that continues throughout life. Once the reactions to negative feelings become a way of life, the child's definitions of normal, comfort, and love are set. It feels right to continue the cycle and the associated family traditions. It's a difficult situation to extract yourself from, and taking care of your own problems is a great start, but not enough to end an unhealthy relationship with food. When you think you have a handle on your reactions and actions, you are not by any means "cured." There are others in your life who are involved, and that's where it gets tricky.

Solutions and Support

I f you are truly ready and have made the decision to tackle your particular problems with eating, you've already taken the first and biggest step forward. The second step is understanding how family and other people affect your diet and exercise lifestyle. You may already recognize that the people in your life may be part of the problem, but you have to go further to better understand the complexities of the connections you have to those people if you want to permanently break the cycle.

And if you are wondering when we will discuss "real" solutions to these problems or how many steps are involved, we just covered the two most difficult steps. The willingness to change and acknowledging outside help is essential for any progress or successful outcome. The rest is built upon this foundation.

Identification and Connection

Identifying issues surrounding unhealthy eating habits and connecting their source(s) are the next steps. They will help you reach your goals and they will also help you maintain your results. The key is to stick with it. Many people who begin to understand their unhealthy habits and start to see results congratulate themselves too early for a job well done and usually end up reverting to their old habits. In fact, it is even common for them to use food to reward themselves—usually unhealthy food, or even a lack of food. That's like celebrating with codeine because you kicked your heroin habit! Stopping at any point in the healing process is like stopping important medication from your doctor—your healing will stop, or worse. Just as people who have kicked alcoholism are still alcoholics and people who quit using drugs are still drug addicts, people who have been dysfunctional eaters or have an eating disorder also retain their unhealthy eating tendencies. For alcoholics and drug addicts, they must stay away from their "drug," but you can't give up eating. So how do you get around this dilemma? Since you can't give up food, you must remove its controlling powers by applying your new knowledge and eating for only two reasons: fuel and nutrition. If you learn to treat your emotional pain and discomfort rather than control them with unhealthy eating habits, then you will be one step closer to breaking your own cycle of addiction.

The Addictive Cycles of Eating shows you how feelings of pain and discomfort are part of a continuing cycle. Well, if you want to stop the cycle, all you have to do is pick something in the cycle to stop, right? But what? The addiction? The need for control? Or the discomfort itself? Surprisingly the answer is none of the above.

The truth is, you can never totally rid yourself of these feelings. All feelings and associated memories you have experienced in your lifetime are part of you—simply put, you are part of your past. But you can effectively limit their influence on your behavior now and in the future. And this will free your mind and give you the strength and ability to stop the unhealthy cycle. By dealing directly with the "cues" or situations that trigger your unhealthy eating habits, you can learn to minimize their powerful influ-

> **YOU ARE PART OF YOUR PAST.**

ences on your feelings and emotions. In fact, you may find that some of these cues that come from other people and cause reactive emotions are usually misinterpretations taken out of context—or not actually as "real" as your mind sees them. Only the emotions that result from these cues are truly real. This isn't an easy task at first, but you can master it by concentrating on two things: identification and connection.

Step One

Identify the feelings that make you want to turn to food as soon as they occur, and try to record as many details about your feelings as possible. Focus on the feeling you are having at the moment you crave something unhealthy or when you find yourself in the middle of your unhealthy eating habits. Then examine the food (quantity and quality), date, time, people, situation, and any other associated details that are a part of these patterns. Use your BOK Journal ⬚ to record your emotions and the associated details. With time, you will notice consistent patterns.

This is an important step. Just the act of recognizing your patterns will help disrupt, slow, and eventually stop the otherwise automatic unhealthy eating habit cycle.

Step Two

Try to hold on to the feelings. After you have identified a feeling and all of its associated details, don't try to force them away. If it is pain, discomfort, anxiety, depression, fear, anger, shame, guilt, or even euphoria or warm, happy feelings, don't try to fight them, immediately dismiss them, or ignore them. Whether it's a few minutes or a few hours, allow the feelings to set their own time schedule. Instinctively, you will probably want to avoid or ignore uncomfortable emotions and feelings. But even that reaction is a part of the problem. Allowing yourself to feel negative or bad feelings is an important step. Then allow yourself to do whatever you normally would do with food in association with that feeling. You will be using this experience to identify an unhealthy eating habit that results from a particular feeling—and then learn from it. Just don't forget to do the same thing with happy feelings that bring about unhealthy eating habits, too. It might be frustrating at first but keep at it.

Step Three

Now connect both the negative or positive feelings and the unhealthy eating habits you have identified with past and present memories and experiences in your lifetime. While you are having feelings that bring about your unhealthy eating habits, think back to similar situations that made you feel the same way. Try to remember who else may have been involved with the feeling. If it's a painful memory (with or without family) or happy celebration or anything you can actually describe, you have made a connection. There may be more than one connection or more than one feeling, so add them to your journal and continue the exercise until you have identified and made connections to as many emotions as possible. This will help you recognize the source(s) of the problem. This connecting information will begin to disconnect you from the cycle and remove its control over your eating habits. It is also valuable if you are involved with proven self-help programs and it's vital to any health professional you may be working with to help you move forward in the healing process.

Most people find that it is difficult to perform these steps on their own, objectively, and without personal bias, so initially a doctor, therapist, or counselor may have to help you identify your emotions and make those critical connections. Again, do whatever works for you, but the goal for all paths on this journey is to eventually have the ability to make the identification and connection on your own every time these feelings arise.

Once you have mastered the identification and connection, try not to jump to conclusions or assume you have all of the answers. These techniques I have outlined are the key steps, but keep an open mind since there are other aspects of the cycle to explore and master. For example, is a person in your life who is trying to "help" you contributing to your discomfort and, by association, your eating disorder? Or do people in your life sometimes unknowingly say things, or give you cues, that connect you with another painful situation from your past? You may misinterpret their comments because of the old connections that remain in your brain that continue to operate unconsciously. Often, others in your life honestly do not realize that their words and actions trigger these cues and contribute to your problems. It takes time to realize and accept these situations before you can think clearly and act appropriately.

Stick with it since these identifying and connecting steps are not only vital for breaking unhealthy cycles but will help clarify a very difficult hurdle (fault). Then you will be ready for your healthiest state of mind and the key to your long-term success. But before I spoil the surprise, let's learn a little bit about the machine that will take you there.

> THESE IDENTIFYING AND CONNECTING STEPS ARE CRUCIAL TO YOUR LONG-TERM SUCCESS.

The Brain: It's Just Another Machine You Can Repair

It is noon on any day in Anywhere, U.S.A., and Anyone, who has been on a diet for some time, is thinking about their favorite food. As usual, Brain Stem, the primitive instigator, is turning up the temptation.

"We've suffered too long on this diet," Brain Stem whines. "It's time to celebrate and reward ourselves for all the weight we lost this week."

Evilly, he turns on the image-maker. A thick, juicy burger, golden fries, and an ice cold cola appear in the mind's eye, instantly driving Taste Buds, who has been patiently awaiting attention, plain crazy.

Brain Stem's more evolved counterpart, Frontal Brain, scoffs back, "Hey, weren't you the one lodging complaints about tight clothes and being tired after meals just a few weeks ago? You hypocrite!"

Taste Buds, suddenly feeling a loss of control, speaks up: "Just this once! We'll skip the fries!"

"That'll be a first," snipes Brain Stem.

Good-intentioned Frontal Brain ignores the comment and calls for rational thought. "But that combination is 1000 calories, 350 calories from fat alone!"

"Give us a break, you fun-hating psycho!" thunders Brain Stem. "A big run after work will burn up the calories. And tomorrow we'll go back to salad, tofu, and no carbs."

"Hey, you know darn well I don't expect us to eat like that," Frontal Brain counters. "And we all know that the kind of food you want will make us feel too heavy to move for hours."

Suddenly emotional mid-brain erupts, "I was getting depressed by your argument, but now you guys are giving me anxiety too! You better take it down a notch, Forebrain, before I have a meltdown and give all the control to Brain Stem."

Brain Stem is just dying for the burger and seizes his chance to play the sympathy card. "Pu-leeease," he says with a whimper.

Frustrated, Frontal Brain reverts to sarcasm: "I have a great idea! Let's pretend we really are intelligent mammals, avoid the burger AND the run. The choice to eat healthier food instead of that greasy meal removes those extra calories instantly. And wouldn't it be nice to spend the evening doing something much more fun than trying to run off those extra calories?"

Sound familiar?

The fully developed brain runs like a sophisticated computer. And like most computers, certain parts are more important than others for performance, and some parts are dependent on others in order to perform at all (Click on the animated tutorial "Welcome to the machine" on the web site homepage to see how it works).

The brain is really just a layered organ of evolution. The most primitive part lies at the base of the skull (the brain stem), and the more advanced sections ascend upward and outward, ending with the most advanced, frontal part of the brain, or forebrain (cerebral cortex). Somewhere in the middle are the areas involved with memory and emotions. This is where unhealthy cycles hide. And some cycles are so powerful they can disrupt your entire thought process. For example, if you turn off a table lamp, it stops the electrical current in the lamp's cord and bulb. The same thing happens in the current in your brain when you are upset, stressed, or scared.

The brain's midsection offers electrical connections between the lower brain stem and the upper brain cortex, where all advanced thinking takes place. As quick as a flick of a light switch, certain emotions can overload our midbrain or paralyze the natural "current of thought." Not only is the current or flow paralyzed, but our usual intelligent reactions are paralyzed too, and we act on dysfunctional brain patterns like any other neurological disorder.

> CERTAIN EMOTIONS CAN OVERLOAD OUR MIDBRAIN OR PARALYZE THE NATURAL FLOW OF THE "THINKING CURRENT."

A great example of a paralyzed midbrain is forgetfulness. Do you ever have trouble remembering something (such as someone's name) when you're put on the spot, stressed, or pressured to remember? Everyone does! Until the situation disappears or you switch to another thought, the current of thought that carries the information you need will be blocked. After the block (stress, heightened emotions, or other disruptive feelings) is removed or has passed, the flow of thought returns and the "remembered" information is able to reach your outer brain and pass to the areas that control speech. Suddenly, what you couldn't remember just spills out of your mouth.

THE CURRENT OF THOUGHT

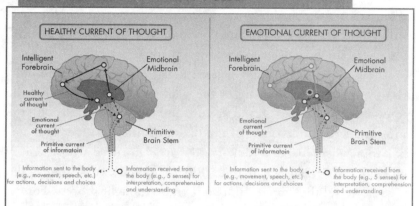

*Stress and emotions that originate in your mind affect the midbrain and can disrupt the normal current of thought—a disruption that can block the forebrain from making healthy, intelligent decisions and choices (solid line), leaving the brain stem's primitive instincts in control based upon more emotional decisions and choices (dashed line). Information that is received from and sent to your body (dotted line) is also affected by stress and emotions. Understanding or interpreting information (from your five senses) as well as the resultant actions (movement, speech, etc.) produced by your decisions and choices all depend upon which path your current of thought takes.

Dysfunctional eating habits and eating disorders involve feelings, emotions, and memories that disrupt the current of thought, too. Not only are our emotions confusing the signals and sending the wrong information to higher areas, they also often block signals altogether. Thus, many decisions or reactions are made with the only machinery available—the machinery in the lower brain stem. This means that all of the basic survival instincts and reward cycles in the more primitive parts of the brain end up affecting most of the decisions associated with food during times of stress, pain, anger, shame, guilt, or sadness as well as euphoria or extreme happiness. Meanwhile, the dysfunctional tools that govern discomfort, addiction, and control are building unhealthy cycles, since the blockage of information prevents the more advanced logical current of thought (forebrain) from making intelligent decisions. Without treatment the unhealthy cycles automatically function within the lower areas of the brain stem and continue to shape our lives based on their primitive reality.

You can' just flip anther switch or quickly fix this either. Correcting this problem requires a rewiring or "bypassing" of your current of thought to the more advanced areas of the brain, the only area capable of making logical—that is, healthy—decisions. To do this, you must first, and most importantly, accept the fact that you can't completely disconnect from your old memories, emotions, and issues with food. You simply cannot remove them.

Like a blocked artery in a heart, you must bypass the problem and reconnect to a healthy area. In the brain, the process is slightly different than in the heart because, unlike the blocked arteries, those old dysfunctional pathways can always open up again. If they do, applying the techniques of action, reaction, identification, and connection

> YOU SIMPLY CANNOT REMOVE THEM [ISSUES WITH FOOD] ... YOU MUST BYPASS THE PROBLEM AND RECONNECT TO A HEALTHY PATTERN.

will keep the healthy bypass open and dysfunctional pathways closed. Once this process is set in motion, you will continue to make the positive decisions that will create new, healthy cycles and continue your healthy current of thought. But how do you keep the unhealthy pathways closed and the new, healthy cycles and pathways open?

Do Whatever It Takes

Once you have identified the origin of your feelings, their connections, and their associated eating habits, you will begin to understand that food (or lack of it) won't make anything better. And after a few attempts at bypassing the unhealthy cycles embedded in your mind using these tools, you'll realize that you can't do it all on your own. The key to success is to want help, to find help, and to accept help. In this mental arena, the core message of Body of Knowledge could not be more important. Your life and unique situations require an individualized treatment plan, and as you make changes, your treatment plan will need to change too. Your success depends on maintaining an open mind, a willingness to try new things, and most importantly a willingness to keep trying and to surround yourself with people who have similar ideals.

After years of practicing medicine, I have figured out the difference between being a good doctor and good doctoring: *do whatever it takes*. When it comes to personal matters, both physical and mental, there is no single solution that is best for everyone. Some will work for you and others won't. Some may work now, but not six months from now. Whether it's traditional medicine, acupuncture, herbal therapy, meditation, religious practice, or just venting frustrations, whatever cures or heads the patient in the right direction is the right treatment.

There are great doctors, counselors, self-help books, videos, DVDs, long-term multi-disciplinary treatment centers, and everything in between to choose from in this day and age. But where do you start? You have already have—by reading this section in the book. You have taken important steps in gaining self-knowledge and self-responsibility for your own heath. In fact, all forms of treatment are useless without your input, and understanding how to gather information about your behavior and emotions is critical. Investigation into your lifestyle and past history is paramount, and who is better qualified to do that than you! "Self-help" is the key to success in all treatment programs.

Another key to your success is recognizing that good eating habits and fitness will be an integral part of your lifestyle, and that you must truly understand this lifestyle change before you can adopt it. You have learned in this book that your mind and body must work together. The healthy eating habits and exercises you have read about are necessary to start, support, and finish your treatment.

You have also learned about the steps you can take to begin to recognize any personal issues that you may have. Now you know that actions, reactions, identification, and connection expose the discomfort and pain that control your particular problems. The next important step is sharing this information with anyone who is a part of your life—that means your family, your significant other, and closest friends. If you want to make any healthy change permanent, the people in your life will have to change, too. And how can they change if you don't let them know how and why you have changed? It may not be easy, but sharing your particular information is crucial to permanently breaking the cycle.

No Fault Zone

Overcoming the all-important hurdle of creating and maintaining healthy cycles and associated pathways of thought involves one more step, which is redirecting your emotions to reach the most important and healthiest state of mind: *forgiveness*. At some point, you must move beyond the need to blame others or yourself for your current situation. In essence, your particular problems are really nobody's "fault." Not many people wake up each morning and consciously set out to make you miserable so they can stick around to wallow in it. Again, they often do not know that they are negatively contributing to your emotional state of mind.

Forgiving whoever or whatever you feel caused your unhealthy, addictive cycles is a critical step for removing the effects of the emotions, feelings, pain, and discomfort—the true driving forces behind your particular difficulties. No blame and fault, no cause and effect, no action and reaction, no addiction, and therefore no more unhealthy eating habits. Simply put, forgiveness removes fault, which removes others involved with an unhealthy current of thought. For it to work, however, forgiveness must be truly felt, not forced. It is a required emotional duty in order to permanently break the cycle.

And don't discount the other part of this process: forgiving *yourself*. It is an important step because taking care of your needs (necessary in order to make permanent, healthy changes) requires truly feeling that you have done nothing wrong and feeling that your needs are as important as others'. In fact, forgiving yourself is a requirement for maintaining forgiveness of others.

Another important factor is a healthy awareness of others and their life scenarios. Too much focus on your own needs may not only create another unhealthy cycle but remove your ability to see that others in your life have similar problems and may need help too. What if they are paralyzed by addictive cycles and experience the same pain and discomfort as you? Once you take the spotlight off of your specific feelings for a moment and try to understand why those in your life do the things they do, you create the opportunity for feelings of

> FORGIVENESS REMOVES FAULT.

empathy for them, which goes hand in hand with true forgiveness. With awareness and practice of all the parameters discussed here, you can create a whole new cycle—one that heals all.

> ## GETTING TO FORGIVENESS: THE HEALTHIEST STATE OF MIND
>
> There are many techniques designed to identify, connect, and share information about the unhealthy cycles that affect our well-being, but all include certain milestones. Here are some steps to consider when confronting issues that involve the people in your life.
>
> - Identify the pain and discomfort by expressing how bad it makes you feel, even if only to yourself.
> - Connect the life situations (past and present verbal, emotional, physical, or sexual abuse) with these feelings.
> - Envision the person or people involved as you are feeling the pain and discomfort.
> - See the new reality that they also experience the same pain and discomfort as you.
> - Accept the fact that they and everyone else in their lives are caught in the same cycle.
> - Feel empathy for them, since you know how bad the experiences and emotions have made you personally feel.
> - Share the identifications, connections, and other information with those who are involved with your unhealthy cycle.
> - Forgive all those who are involved with your unhealthy cycle.
> - Make yourself available to others and be open to intimacy.
> - Set personal boundaries and maintain them when you introduce your new, healthy lifestyle to others.
> - Make yourself available for discussion and listen to all opinions and rebuttals.

A Little Extra Help

For many of you, shifting to a healthy reality can be very hard. You could be held back by something as serious as physical or sexual abuse, by verbal and emotional abuse, a general low self-esteem, or by simply not having a clue as to the source of your issues. If at first you can't shake feelings of fear, anger, shame, and guilt, or embrace empathy and forgiveness, don't give up. That is what your doctor or counselor is there for—to help you through these obstacles and then to help you do it on your own. Think of counseling as a personal trainer for your mind. Some of us may need just a few sessions to catch on while others may need intimate, prolonged coaching. Counseling at any level is always a positive move forward. There are many qualified counselors, therapists, psychologists, social workers, or psychiatrists available who are able and willing to help. There is no mystery to their scientifically proven techniques, and there is definitely no reason to be embarrassed about using their services.

If you have followed all of the advice in Body of Knowledge and are still struggling with your health, weight management, fitness, or other personal issues, then it is likely you do need to seek professional help. And if you have the symptoms of any eating disorder, then you need to seek professional help immediately. Self-help alone or within a family setting can work for some minor issues, but only if you and all involved focus on critical problems and continue working to reach a healthy solution.

It can be hard to maintain a healthy current of thought while experiencing the very cycles you are trying to break though. Unhealthy arguments, avoiding issues, displaying false emotions, and excluding key people can make it worse. Counseling, on the other hand, offers non-biased intervention by a trained professional. Be it a one-on-one session or a group setting, these trained referees know what it takes to cultivate healthy habits.

As you can tell, most of your efforts to deal with the root causes of unhealthy eating habits and problems with weight management will be centered on family and social issues. I am by no means suggesting that you round up your parents, grandparents, siblings, uncles, aunts, cousins, friends, and coworkers and hold them hostage while you hammer out a list of painful issues. The process is as unique as each individual, but the past is where you will find the majority of the reasons behind your particular problems. Don't go overboard though and make another common mistake by trying to "make up for the past"—please focus only on today and on moving forward. In true Body of Knowledge fashion, I would like you to simply take the information you have gained in this section, apply it to any situation you choose, and then see what happens. Of course my goal is to help you stick with it until any unhealthy physical or mental situation is resolved, but it's time for you to take over and start using your Body of Knowledge.

GROUP THERAPY: WHY IT WORKS

Group cognitive behavioral therapy (CBT) can guide individuals through the thoughts, feelings, and environmental/social conditions associated with dysfunctional eating and lifestyle behaviors in a group setting. It can be effective beyond expectations.

The counselor probes habitual behaviors, perceived influences, and barriers to corrective action as part of group discussion. Participants discuss their coping attempts with the group and the counselor discusses how improvements might be made. Technical terms such as self-monitoring (self-recognition of problems), stimulus control (management of unhealthy "cues" and addictions), contingency management (regulation of interactions like dependency and co-dependency), and use of social support (support from family, friends, work, school, etc.) are basic to this approach. In the end, everyone involved is held responsible and accountable for his or her involvement in creating the perfect environment for providing lasting solutions to immediate and future problems.

Just the Beginning

This may be the end of the book but it's just the beginning of your journey. Now it's your turn to take your newfound knowledge and put it to work, for yourself and the people you love. What you eat, how you eat, how often you eat, and how well you exercise will change your life for the better. I hope that you will start putting as much energy into your health as you do work or play or family. Remember, if you don't take care of *you*, you can't take care of anyone else.

I encourage you to keep this book handy and refer to your notes and the pages you have marked. I hope this will become the most dog-eared book in your house. And thanks to the miracle of the internet, you can continue your lifestyle lessons on the web site, which is also designed to change as you change. Log on and let me know how you are doing. What is working or not working for you and for others in your part of the world? Do you have any suggestions or ideas that could make your experience better? I love to hear from patients and readers.

Mastering health and fitness is my gift to you, and now it is yours to share with those you care about the most. Good luck and enjoy one of the few gifts that truly keeps on giving—a Body of Knowledge.

Bibliography

Introduction

Bowerman, S., M. Bellman, P. Saltsman, D. Garvey, K. Pimstone, et. al. "Implementation of a primary care physician network obesity management program." *Obes Res* 9, Suppl. (2001):321S–325S.

Lyznicki, J.M., D.C. Young, J.A., Riggs, R.M. Davis. "Obesity: assessment and management in primary care." *Am Fam Physician* 63, no. 11 (2001): 2185–96.

Sturm, R. "The effects of obesity, smoking, and drinking on medical problems and costs." *Health Affairs* 21, Issue 2 (2002): 245–253.

Part 1: Welcome to the Machine

Astrup, A., T. Meinert Larsen, and A. Harper. "Atkins and Other Low-Carbohydrate Diets: Hoax or an Effective Tool for Weight Loss?" *Lancet* 364, no. 9437 (2004): 897–899.

Bertakis, K. D., and R. Azari. "Obesity and the Use of Health Care Services." *Obes Res* 13, no. 2 (2005): 372–379.

Byers, T., M. Nestle, A. McTiernan, C. Doyle, A. Currie-Williams, et al. "American Cancer Society Guidelines on Nutrition and Physical Activity for Cancer Prevention: Reducing the Risk of Cancer with Healthy Food Choices and Physical Activity." *CA Cancer J Clin* 52, no. 2 (2002): 92–119.

Calle, E. E., C. Rodriguez, K. Walker-Thurmond, and M. J. Thun. "Overweight, Obesity, and Mortality from Cancer in a Prospectively Studied Cohort of U.S. Adults." *N Engl J Med* 348, no. 17 (2003): 1625–1638.

"Diet, Nutrition and the Prevention of Chronic Diseases." *World Health Organ Tech Rep Ser* 916 (2003): i–viii, 1–149, back cover.

Elliot, D. L., and L. Goldberg. "Nutrition and Exercise." *Med Clin North Am* 69, no. 1 (1985): 71–82.

Finkelstein, E. A., I. C. Fiebelkorn, and G. Wang. "National Medical Spending Attributable to Overweight and Obesity: How Much, and Who's Paying?" *Health Aff* (Millwood) Suppl (2003): W3-219–W3-226.

Heggie, S. J., M. J. Wiseman, G. J. Cannon, L. M. Miles, R. L. Thompson, et al. "Defining the State of Knowledge with Respect to Food, Nutrition, Physical Activity, and the Prevention of Cancer." *J Nutr* 133, no. 11 Suppl 1 (2003).

Jackson, Y., W. H. Dietz, C. Sanders, L. J. Kolbe, J. J. Whyte, et al. "Summary of the 2000 Surgeon General's Listening Session: Toward a National Action Plan on Overweight and Obesity." *Obes Res* 10, no. 12 (2002): 1299–1305.

Jeffery, R. W., A. Drewnowski, L.H. Epstein, A.J. Stunkard, G.T. Wilson, R.R. Wing, et al. "Long-Term Maintenance of Weight Loss: Current Status." *Health Psychology: Official Journal of the Division of Health Psychology, American Psychological Association* 19 no. 1 Suppl (2000): 5–16.

Key, T. J., N. E. Allen, E. A. Spencer, and R. C. Travis. "The Effect of Diet on Risk of Cancer." *Lancet* 360, no. 9336 (2002): 861–868.

Lang, A., & E.S. Froelicher. "Management of Overweight and Obesity in Adults: Behavioral Intervention for Long-Term Weight Loss and Maintenance." *Eur J of Card Nur: J of the Working Group on Card Nur of the Eur Society of Card* 5 no. 2 (2006):102–114.

Lowe, M. R. "Self-Regulation of Energy Intake in the Prevention and Treatment of Obesity: Is It Feasible?" *Obes Res* 11 Suppl (2003): 44S–59S.

Lubin, F., A. Lusky, A. Chetrit, and R. Dankner. "Lifestyle and Ethnicity Play a Role in All-Cause Mortality." *J Nutr* 133, no. 4 (2003): 1180–1185.

Peeters, A., J. J. Barendregt, F. Willekens, J. P. Mackenbach, A. Al Mamun, and L. Bonneux. "Obesity in Adulthood and Its Consequences for Life Expectancy: A Life-Table Analysis." *Ann Intern Med* 138, no. 1 (2003): 24–32.

Part 2: Food and Eating Habits

Allman-Farinelli, M. A., K. Gomes, E. J. Favaloro, and P. Petocz. "A Diet Rich in High-Oleic-Acid Sunflower Oil Favorably Alters Low-Density Lipoprotein Cholesterol, Triglycerides, and Factor Vii Coagulant Activity." *J Am Diet Assoc* 105, no. 7 (2005): 1071–1079.

Altman, T. A. *FDA and USDA Nutrition Labeling Guide: Decision Diagrams, Checklists, and Regulations.* (2002) Boca Raton: CRC Press.

Asano, T., T. Ogihara, H. Katagiri, H. Sakoda, H. Ono, et al. "Glucose Transporter and Na+/Glucose cotransporter as Molecular Targets of Anti-diabetic Drugs." *Cur Med Chem* 11 (2004): 2717–2724.

Ball, S. D., K. R. Keller, L. J. Moyer-Mileur, Y. W. Ding, D. Donaldson, and W. D. Jackson. "Prolongation of Satiety after Low Versus Moderately High Glycemic Index Meals in Obese Adolescents." *Pediatrics* 111, no. 3 (2003): 488–494.

Barfull, A., C. Garriga, A. Tauler, and J. M. Planas. "Regulation of Sglt1 Expression in Response to Na(+) Intake." *Am J Physiol Regul Integr Comp Physiol* 282, no. 3 (2002): R738–R743.

Brynes, A. E., J. Adamson, A. Dornhorst, and G. S. Frost. "The Beneficial Effect of a Diet with Low Glycaemic Index on 24 H Glucose Profiles in Healthy Young People as Assessed by

Continuous Glucose Monitoring." *Br J Nutr* 93, no. 2 (2005): 179–182.

Cheng, C., C. Graziani, and J. J. Diamond. "Cholesterol-Lowering Effect of the Food for Heart Nutrition Education Program." *J Am Diet Assoc* 104, no. 12 (2004): 1868–1872.

Cordain, L., J. B. Miller, S. B. Eaton, N. Mann, S. H. Holt, and J. D. Speth. "Plant-Animal Subsistence Ratios and Macro-nutrient Energy Estimations in Worldwide Hunter-Gatherer Diets." *Am J Clin Nutr* 71, no. 3 (2000): 682–692.

da Costa Lima, N. K., F. B. Lima, E. A. dos Santos, M. M. Okamo-to, D. H. Matsushita, et al. "Chronic Salt Overload Increases Blood Pressure and Improves Glucose Metabolism without Changing Insulin Sensitivity." *Am J Hypertens* 10, no. 7 Pt 1 (1997): 720–727.

de Lauzon-Guillain, B., A. Basdevant, M. Romon, J. Karlsson, J.M. Borys, et al. "Is Restrained Eating a Risk Factor for Weight Gain in a General Population?" *Am J Clin Nutr* 2006; 83: 132–138.

Drewnowski, A., and M. R. Greenwood. "Cream and Sugar: Human Preferences for High-Fat Foods." *Physiol Behav* 30, no. 4 (1983): 629–633.

Dyer, J., P. J. Barker, and S. P. Shirazi-Beechey. "Nutrient Regulation of the Intestinal Na+/Glucose Co-Transporter (Sglt1) Gene Expression." *Biochem Biophys Res Commun* 230, no. 3 (1997): 624–629.

Ebbeling, C. B., M. M. Leidig, K. B. Sinclair, L. G. Seger-Ship-pee, H. A. Feldman, and D. S. Ludwig. "Effects of an Ad Libitum Low-Glycemic Load Diet on Cardiovascular Disease Risk Factors in Obese Young Adults." *Am J Clin Nutr* 81, no. 5 (2005): 976–982.

Ehrenkranz, J. R., N. G. Lewis, C. Ronald Kahn, and J. Roth. "Phlorizin: A Review." *Diabetes Metab Res Rev* 21, no. 1 (2005): 31–38.

Epstein, L. H., C. C. Gordy, H. A. Raynor, M. Beddome, C. K. Kilanowski, and R. Paluch. "Increasing Fruit and Vegetable Intake and Decreasing Fat and Sugar Intake in Families at Risk for Childhood Obesity." *Obes Res* 9, no. 3 (2001): 171–178.

Farshchi, H. R., M. A. Taylor, and I. A. Macdonald. "Beneficial Metabolic Effects of Regular Meal Frequency on Dietary Thermogenesis, Insulin Sensitivity, and Fasting Lipid Profiles in Healthy Obese Women." *Am J Clin Nutr* 81, no. 1 (2005): 16–24.

Flatt, J. P. "Macronutrient Composition and Food Selection." *Obes Res* 9 Suppl 4 (2001): 256S–262S.

Freeland-Graves, J., and S. Nitzke. "Position of the American Dietetic Association: Total Diet Approach to Communicating Food and Nutrition Information." *J Am Diet Assoc* 102, no. 1 (2002): 100–108.

Fuenmayor, N., E. Moreira, and L. X. Cubeddu. "Salt Sensitivity Is Associated with Insulin Resistance in Essential Hypertension." *Am J Hypertens* 11, no. 4 Pt 1 (1998): 397–402.

Gerhard, G. T., A. Ahmann, K. Meeuws, M. P. McMurry, P. B. Duell, and W. E. Connor. "Effects of a Low-Fat Diet Compared with Those of a High-Monounsaturated Fat Diet on Body Weight, Plasma Lipids and Lipoproteins, and Glycemic Control in Type 2 Diabetes." *Am J Clin Nutr* 80, no. 3 (2004): 668–673.

Gillen, L. J., L. C. Tapsell, C. S. Patch, A. Owen, and M. Batterham. "Structured Dietary Advice Incorporating Walnuts Achieves Optimal Fat and Energy Balance in Patients with Type 2 Diabetes Mellitus." *J Am Diet Assoc* 105, no. 7 (2005): 1087–1096.

Gross, L. S., L. Li, E. S. Ford, and S. Liu. "Increased Consumption of Refined Carbohydrates and the Epidemic of Type 2 Diabetes in the United States: An Ecologic Assessment." *Am J Clin Nutr* 79, no. 5 (2004): 774–779.

Haslam, D. W., & W.P.T. James. "Obesity." Lancet 366 no. 9492 (2005):1197- 1209.

Hetherington, M. M., F. Cameron, D. J. Wallis, and L. M. Pirie. "Stimulation of Appetite by Alcohol." *Physiol Behav* 74, no. 3 (2001): 283–289.

Hollenberg, N.K. "The Influence of Dietary Sodium on Blood Pressure." *J Am Coll Nutr* Vol. 25 Suppl 3 (2006): 240S–246S.

Institute of Medicine (U.S.), & Standing Committee on the Scientific Evaluation of Dietary Reference Intakes. "Dietary Reference Intakes for Energy, Carbohydrate, Fiber, Fat, Fatty Acids, Cholesterol, Protein and Amino Acids" (2002) Washington, D.C: National Academy Press.

Jenkins, D. J., T. M. Wolever, V. Vuksan, F. Brighenti, S. C. Cunnane, et al. "Nibbling Versus Gorging: Metabolic Advantages of Increased Meal Frequency." *N Engl J Med* 321, no. 14 (1989): 929–934.

Kretser, A. J. "The New Dietary Reference Intakes in Food Labeling: The Food Industry's Perspective." *The Am J of Clin Nutr* 83 no. 5 (2006): 1231S–1234s.

Lapointe, J. Y., M. P. Gagnon, D. G. Gagnon, and P. Bissonnette. "Controversy Regarding the Secondary Active Water Transport Hypothesis." *Biochem Cell Biol* 80, no. 5 (2002): 525–533.

Ledikwe, J. H., H.M. Blanck, L. Kettel Khan, M.K. Serdula, J.D. Seymour, B.C. Tohill, et al. "Dietary Energy Density is Associated with Energy Intake and Weight Status in US Adults." *The Am J of Clin Nutr*, 83 no. 6 (2006): 1362–1368.

Ledikwe, J. H., J. A. Ello-Martin, and B. J. Rolls. "Portion Sizes and the Obesity Epidemic." *J Nutr* 135, no. 4 (2005): 905–909.

Lejeune, M. P., E. M. Kovacs, and M. S. Westerterp-Plantenga. "Additional Protein Intake Limits Weight Regain after Weight Loss in Humans." *Br J Nutr* 93, no. 2 (2005): 281–289.

Li, Z., S. Lamon-Fava, J. Otvos, A. H. Lichtenstein, W. Velez-Carrasco, J. R. McNamara, et al. "Fish Consumption Shifts

Lipoprotein Subfractions to a Less Atherogenic Pattern in Humans." *J Nutr* 134, no. 7 (2004): 1724–1728.

Mate, A., A. Barfull, A.M. Hermosa, L. Gomez-Amores, C.M. Vazquez, et al. "Regulation of Sodium-Glucose Cotransporter SGLT1 in the Intestine of Hypertensive Rats." *Am J Physiol Regulatory Integrative Comp Physiol* 291 (2006): 760–767.

McCarty, M. F. "The Origins of Western Obesity: A Role for Animal Protein?" *Med Hypotheses* 54, no. 3 (2000): 488–494.

McCrory, M. A., V. M. Suen, and S. B. Roberts. "Biobehavioral Influences on Energy Intake and Adult Weight Gain." *J Nutr* 132, no. 12 (2002).

Meinild, A., D. A. Klaerke, D. D. Loo, E. M. Wright, and T. Zeuthen. "The Human Na+-Glucose Cotransporter is a Molecular Water Pump." *J Physiol* 508 (Pt 1) (1998): 15–21.

Merchant, A. T., F. B. Hu, D. Spiegelman, W. C. Willett, E. B. Rimm, and A. Ascherio. "Dietary Fiber Reduces Peripheral Arterial Disease Risk in Men." *J Nutr* 133, no. 11 (2003): 3658–3663.

Murphy, S. P., and R. K. Johnson. "The Scientific Basis of Recent Us Guidance on Sugars Intake." *Am J Clin Nutr* 78, no. 4 (2003): 827S–833S.

Nunoi, K., K. Yasuda, T. Adachi, Y. Okamoto, N. Shihara, et al. "Beneficial Effect of T-1095, a Selective Inhibitor of Renal Na+-Glucose Cotransporters, on Metabolic Index and Insulin Secretion in Spontaneously Diabetic GK Rats." *Clin Exp Pharm and Phys* 29 (2002): 386–390.

Oku, A., K. Ueta, M. Nawano, K. Arakawa, T. Kano-Ishihara, et al. "Antidiabetic Effect of T-1095, an Inhibitor of Na+-Glucose Cotransporter, in Neonatally Streptozotocin-Treated Rats." *Eur J Pharm* 391 (2000): 183–192.

Parr, T. "Insulin Exposure and Aging Theory." *Gerontology* 43, no. 3 (1997): 182–200.

Pasman, W. J., V. M. Blokdijk, F. M. Bertina, W. P. Hopman, and H. F. Hendriks. "Effect of Two Breakfasts, Different in Carbohydrate Composition, on Hunger and Satiety and Mood in Healthy Men." *Int J Obes Relat Metab Disord* 27, no. 6 (2003): 663–8.

Pittler, M. H., and E. Ernst. "Dietary Supplements for Body-Weight Reduction: A Systematic Review." *Am J Clin Nutr* 79, no. 4 (2004): 529–536.

Raben, A., T. H. Vasilaras, A. C. Moller, and A. Astrup. "Sucrose Compared with Artificial Sweeteners: Different Effects on Ad Libitum Food Intake and Body Weight after 10 Wk of Supplementation in Overweight Subjects." *Am J Clin Nutr* 76, no. 4 (2002): 721–729.

Reddy, M. B., and M. Love. "The Impact of Food Processing on the Nutritional Quality of Vitamins and Minerals." *Adv Exp Med Biol* 459 (1999): 99–106.

Resnick, L. M., M. Barbagallo, L. J. Dominguez, J. M. Veniero, J. P. Nicholson, and R. K. Gupta. "Relation of Cellular Potassium to Other Mineral Ions in Hypertension and Diabetes." *Hypertension* 38, no. 3 Pt 2 (2001): 709–712.

Rissanen, T. H., S. Voutilainen, J. K. Virtanen, B. Venho, M. Vanharanta, et al. "Low Intake of Fruits, Berries and Vegetables Is Associated with Excess Mortality in Men: The Kuopio Ischaemic Heart Disease Risk Factor (Kihd) Study." *J Nutr* 133, no. 1 (2003): 199–204.

Rocchini, A.P. "Obesity Hypertension, Salt Sensitivity and Insulin Resistance." *Nutr Metab Cardiov Dis* 10, 5 (2000): 287–94.

Rolls, B. J., L. S. Roe, and J. S. Meengs. "Salad and Satiety: Energy Density and Portion Size of a First-Course Salad Affect Energy Intake at Lunch." *J Am Diet Assoc* 104, no. 10 (2004): 1570–1576.

Speechly, D. P., and R. Buffenstein. "Appetite Dysfunction in Obese Males: Evidence for Role of Hyperinsulinaemia in Passive Overconsumption with a High Fat Diet." *Eur J Clin Nutr* 54, no. 3 (2000): 225–233.

Speechly, D. P., G. G. Rogers, and R. Buffenstein. "Acute Appetite Reduction Associated with an Increased Frequency of Eating in Obese Males." *Int J Obes Relat Metab Disord* 23, no. 11 (1999): 1151–1159.

Stubbs, R. J. "Peripheral Signals Affecting Food Intake." *Nutrition* 15, no. 7-8 (1999): 614–625.

Suzuki, M., Y. Kimura, M. Tsushima, and Y. Harano. "Association of Insulin Resistance with Salt Sensitivity and Nocturnal Fall of Blood Pressure." *Hypertension* 35, no. 4 (2000): 864–868.

Sweeney, G., and A. Klip. "Mechanisms and Consequences of the Na+, K+ Pump Regulation by Insulin and Leptin." *Cell Mol Biol* 47-2 (2001): 363–372.

Tholstrup, T., L. I. Hellgren, M. Petersen, S. Basu, E. M. Straarup, et al. "A Solid Dietary Fat Containing Fish Oil Redistributes Lipoprotein Subclasses without Increasing Oxidative Stress in Men." *J Nutr 134*, no. 5 (2004): 1051–1057.

Thorburn, A. W., J. C. Brand, and A. S. Truswell. "Salt and the Glycemic Response." *Br Med J (Clin Res Ed)* 292, no. 6537 (1986): 1697–1699.

Timlin, M. T., and E. J. Parks. "Temporal Pattern of De Novo Lipogenesis in the Postprandial State in Healthy Men." *Am J Clin Nutr* 81, no. 1 (2005): 35–42.

Ueta, K., T. Ishihara, Y. Matsumoto, A. Oku, M. Navano, et al. "Long-term treatment with the Na+ Glucose Cotransporter Inhibitor T-1095 Causes Sustained Improvement in Hyperglycimia in GK Rats." *Life Sciences* 76 (2005): 2655–2668.

Westphal, S., S. Kastner, E. Taneva, A. Leodolter, J. Dierkes, and C. Luley. "Postprandial Lipid and Carbohydrate Responses after the Ingestion of a Casein-Enriched Mixed Meal." *Am J Clin Nutr* 80, no. 2 (2004): 284–290.

Wigertz, K., C. Palacios, L.A. Jackman, B.R. Martin, L.D. McCabe, G.P. McCabe, et al. "Racial Differences in Calcium Retention in Response to Dietary Salt in Adolescent Girls." *The Am J of Clin Nutr* 81 (2005): 845–850.

Zeuthen, T., and N. MacAulay. "Cotransporters as Molecular Water Pumps." *Int Rev Cytol* 215 (2002): 259–284.

Zeuthen, T., A. K. Meinild, D. D. Loo, E. M. Wright, and D. A. Klaerke. "Isotonic Transport by the Na+-Glucose Cotransporter Sglt1 from Humans and Rabbit." *J Physiol* 531, Pt 3 (2001): 631–644.

Part 3: Activity and Exercise

Baker, D., and R. U. Newton. "Acute Effect on Power Output of Alternating an Agonist and Antagonist Muscle Exercise During Complex Training." *J Strength Cond Res* 19, no. 1 (2005): 202–205.

Balabinis, C. P., C. H. Psarakis, M. Moukas, M. P. Vassiliou, and P. K. Behrakis. "Early Phase Changes by Concurrent Endurance and Strength Training." *J Strength Cond Res* 17, no. 2 (2003): 393–401.

Blair, S. N., M. J. LaMonte, and M. Z. Nichaman. "The Evolution of Physical Activity Recommendations: How Much Is Enough?" *Am J Clin Nutr* 79, no. 5 (2004): 913S–920S.

Blix, G. G., and A. G. Blix. "The Role of Exercise in Weight Loss." *Behav Med* 21, no. 1 (1995): 31–39.

Blomstrand, E., J. Eliasson, H.K.R. Karlsson, and R. Kohnke. "Branched-Chain Amino Acids Activate Key Enzymes in Protein Synthesis after Physical Exercise." *J Nutr* 136 (1) (2006): 269S–273S.

Brooks, G. A., N. F. Butte, W. M. Rand, J. P. Flatt, and B. Caballero. "Chronicle of the Institute of Medicine Physical Activity Recommendation: How a Physical Activity Recommendation Came to Be among Dietary Recommendations." *Am J Clin Nutr* 79, no. 5 (2004): 921S–930S.

Byrne, N. M., R. L. Weinsier, G. R. Hunter, R. Desmond, M. A. Patterson, et al. "Influence of Distribution of Lean Body Mass on Resting Metabolic Rate after Weight Loss and Weight Regain: Comparison of Responses in White and Black Women." *Am J Clin Nutr* 77, no. 6 (2003): 1368–1373.

Elliot, D. L., and L. Goldberg. "Nutrition and Exercise." *Med Clin North Am* 69, no.1 (1985): 71–82.

Gilliat-Wimberly, M., M. M. Manore, K. Woolf, P. D. Swan, and S. S. Carroll. "Effects of Habitual Physical Activity on the Resting Metabolic Rates and Body Compositions of Women Aged 35 to 50 Years." *J Am Diet Assoc* 101, no. 10 (2001): 1181–1188.

Goodpaster, B. H., R. R. Wolfe, and D. E. Kelley. "Effects of Obesity on Substrate Utilization During Exercise." *Obes Res* 10, no. 7 (2002): 575–584.

Holcomb, C. A., D. L. Heim, and T. M. Loughin. "Physical Activity Minimizes the Association of Body Fatness with Abdominal Obesity in White, Premenopausal Women: Results from the Third National Health and Nutrition Examination Survey." *J Am Diet Assoc* 104, no. 12 (2004): 1859–1862.

Hunter, G. R., J. P. McCarthy, and M. M. Bamman. "Effects of Resistance Training on Older Adults." *Sports Med* 34, no. 5 (2004): 329–348.

Jakicic, J. M., and A. D. Otto. "Physical Activity Considerations for the Treatment and Prevention of Obesity." *Am J Clin Nutr* 82, no. 1 (2005): 226S–229S.

Jakicic, J. M., R. R. Wing, and C. Winters-Hart. "Relationship of Physical Activity to Eating Behaviors and Weight Loss in Women." *Med Sci Sports Exerc* 34, no. 10 (2002): 1653–1659.

Jeffery, R. W., R. R. Wing, N. E. Sherwood, and D. F. Tate. "Physical Activity and Weight Loss: Does Prescribing Higher Physical Activity Goals Improve Outcome?" *Am J Clin Nutr* 78, no. 4 (2003): 684–689.

Kraemer, W.J., N.A. Ratamess, D.N. French. "Resistance Training for Health and Performance." *Curr Sports Med Rep* 1(3) (2002): 165–171.

Long, S. J., K. Hart, and L. M. Morgan. "The Ability of Habitual Exercise to Influence Appetite and Food Intake in Response to High- and Low-Energy Preloads in Man." *Br J Nutr* 87, no. 5 (2002): 517–523.

Okura, T., Y. Nakata, and K. Tanaka. "Effects of Exercise Intensity on Physical Fitness and Risk Factors for Coronary Heart Disease." *Obes Res* 11, no. 9 (2003): 1131–1139.

Pate, R. R., M. Pratt, S. N. Blair, W. L. Haskell, C. A. Macera, C. Bouchard, et al. "Physical Activity and Public Health. A Recommendation from the Centers for Disease Control and Prevention and the American College of Sports Medicine." *J ama* 273, no. 5 (1995): 402–407.

Pikosky, M. A., P.C. Gaine, W.F. Martin, K.C. Grabarz, A.A. Ferrando, R.R. Wolfe, et al. "Aerobic Exercise Training Increases Skeletal Muscle Protein Turnover in Healthy Adults at Rest." *J of Nutr* 136 (2006): 379-383.

Rhea, M. R., B. A. Alvar, S. D. Ball, and L. N. Burkett. "Three Sets of Weight Training Superior to 1 Set with Equal Intensity for Eliciting Strength." *J Strength Cond Res* 16, no. 4 (2002): 525–529.

Schoeller, D. A., K. Shay, and R. F. Kushner. "How Much Physical Activity Is Needed to Minimize Weight Gain in Previously Obese Women?" *Am J Clin Nutr* 66, no. 3 (1997): 551–556.

Shimomura, Y., Y. Yamamoto, G. Bajotto, J. Sato, T. Murakami, N. Shimomura, et al. "Nutraceutical Effects of Branched-Chain Amino Acids on Skeletal Muscle." *J of Nutr* 136(2) (2006): 529S–532S.

Speakman, J.R., C. Selman. "Physical Activity and Resting Metabolic Rate." *Proc Nutr Soc* 62 (3) (2003): 621–634.

Taaffe, D. R., L. Pruitt, J. Reim, G. Butterfield, and R. Marcus. "Effect of Sustained Resistance Training on Basal Metabolic Rate in Older Women." *J Am Geriatr Soc* 43, no. 5 (1995): 465–471.

Turcotte, L. P. "Role of Fats in Exercise. Types and Quality." *Clin Sports Med* 18, no.3 (1999): 485–498.

Utter, J., D. Neumark-Sztainer, R. Jeffery, and M. Story. "Couch Potatoes or French Fries: Are Sedentary Behaviors Associated with Body Mass Index, Physical Activity, and Dietary Behaviors among Adolescents?" *J Am Diet Assoc* 103, no. 10 (2003): 1298–1305.

Weiss, L. W., L. E. Wood, A. C. Fry, R. B. Kreider, G. E. Relyea, et al. "Strength/Power Augmentation Subsequent to Short-Term Training Abstinence." *J Strength Cond* Res 18, no. 4 (2004): 765–770.

Wilmore, J. H., J. P. Despres, P. R. Stanforth, S. Mandel, T. Rice, et al. "Alterations in Body Weight and Composition Consequent to 20 Wk of Endurance Training: The Heritage Family Study." *Am J Clin Nutr* 70, no. 3 (1999): 346–352.

Wolfe, R. R. "Skeletal Muscle Protein Metabolism and Resistance Exercise." *J of Nutr* 136 (2006): 525S–528S.

Part 4: Putting It All Together

Blass, E. M. "Biological and Environmental Determinants of Childhood Obesity." *Nutr Clin Care* 6, no. 1 (2003): 13–19.

Dalle Grave, R., S. Calugi, E. Molinari, M.L. Petroni, M. Bondi, A. Compare, et al. "Weight Loss Expectations in Obese Patients and Treatment Attrition: An Observational Multicenter Study." *Obesity Research* 13 (2005): 1961–1969.

Dietz, W. H. "The Obesity Epidemic in Young Children. Reduce Television Viewing and Promote Playing." *BMJ* 322, no. 7282 (2001): 313–314.

Hill, J. C., P. C. Smith, and S. E. Meadows. "What Are the Most Effective Interventions to Reduce Childhood Obesity?" *J Fam Pract* 51, no. 10 (2002):891.

Hoelscher, D. M., A. Evans, G. S. Parcel, and S. H. Kelder. "Designing Effective Nutrition Interventions for Adolescents." *J Am Diet Assoc* 102, no. 3 Suppl (2002): S52–S63.

Jenkins, D. J., T. M. Wolever, V. Vuksan, F. Brighenti, S. C. Cunnane, et al. "Nibbling Versus Gorging: Metabolic Advantages of Increased Meal Frequency." *N Engl J Med* 321, no. 14 (1989): 929–934.

Raynor, H. A., C. K. Kilanowski, I. Esterlis, and L. H. Epstein. "A Cost-Analysis of Adopting a Healthful Diet in a Family-Based Obesity Treatment Program." *J Am Diet Assoc* 102, no. 5 (2002): 645–656.

Speechly, D. P., and R. Buffenstein. "Greater Appetite Control Associated with an Increased Frequency of Eating in Lean Males." *Appetite* 33, no. 3 (1999):285–297.

Story, M., D. Neumark-Sztainer, and S. French. "Individual and Environmental Influences on Adolescent Eating Behaviors." *J Am Diet Assoc* 102, no. 3 Suppl (2002): S40–S51.

Utter, J., D. Neumark-Sztainer, R. Jeffery, and M. Story. "Couch Potatoes or French Fries: Are Sedentary Behaviors Associated with Body Mass Index, Physical Activity, and Dietary Behaviors among Adolescents?" *J Am Diet Assoc* 103, no. 10 (2003): 1298–1305.

Part 5: Mind Over Matter

Anderson, S.E., P. Cohen, E.N. Naumova, and A. Must. "Association of Depression and Anxiety Disorders with Weight Change in a Prospective Community-Based Study of Children Followed Up into Adulthood." *Arch Pediatr Adolesc Med* 160(3) (2006): 285–191.

Becker, A. E., S.K. Grinspoon, A. Klibanski, & D.B. Herzog. "Eating disorders." *New England J of Med* 340, no.14 (1999):1092.

Bellisle, F. "Effects of Diet on Behaviour and Cognition in Children." *Br J Nutr* 92 Suppl 2 (2004): S227–S232.

Birch, L. L. "Psychological Influences on the Childhood Diet." *J Nutr* 128, no. 2 Suppl (1998): 407S–410S.

Dietz, W. H. "Health Consequences of Obesity in Youth: Childhood." *Pediatrics* 101 no. 3 (1998): 518.

Foreyt, J. P., and W. S. Poston, 2nd. "What Is the Role of Cognitive-Behavior Therapy in Patient Management?" *Obes Res* 6 Suppl 1 (1998): 18S–22S.

Fox, M. K., B. Devaney, K. Reidy, C. Razafindrakoto, & P. Ziegler. "Relationship Between Portion Size and Energy Intake Among Infants and Toddlers: Evidence of Self-Regulation." *J of the Am Dietetic Association* 106 vol. 1 Suppl 1 (2006): S77–83.

Fulkerson, J. A., D. Neumark-Sztainer, & M. Story. "Adolescent and Parent Views of Family Meals." *J of the Am Dietetic Association* 106 vol. 4 (2006): 526–532.

Gingras, J., J. Fitzpatrick, and L. McCargar. "Body Image of Chronic Dieters: Lowered Appearance Evaluation and Body Satisfaction." *J Am Diet Assoc* 104, no. 10 (2004): 1589–92.

Goodman, E., and R. C. Whitaker. "A Prospective Study of the Role of Depression in the Development and Persistence of Adolescent Obesity." *Pediatrics* 110, no. 3 (2002): 497–504.

Gribble, L. S., G. Falciglia, A. M. Davis, and S. C. Couch. "A Curriculum Based on Social Learning Theory Emphasizing Fruit Exposure and Positive Parent Child-Feeding Strategies: A Pilot Study." *J Am Diet Assoc* 103, no. 1 (2003):100–103.

Halkjaer, J., C. Holst, and T. I. Sorensen. "Intelligence Test Score and Educational Level in Relation to Bmi Changes and Obesity." *Obes Res* 11, no. 10 (2003): 1238–1245.

Hancox, R. J., B. J. Milne, and R. Poulton. "Association between Child and Adolescent Television Viewing and Adult Health: A Longitudinal Birth Cohort Study." *Lancet* 364, no. 9430 (2004): 257–262.

Laessle, R. G., H. Uhl, and B. Lindel. "Parental Influences on Eating Behavior in Obese and Nonobese Preadolescents." *Int J Eat Disord* 30, no. 4 (2001): 447–453.

Latner, J. D., and A. J. Stunkard. "Getting Worse: The Stigmatization of Obese Children." *Obes Res* 11, no. 3 (2003): 452–456.

Leigh Gibson, E. "Emotional Influences on Food Choice: Sensory, Physiological and Psychological Pathways." *Physiology & Behavior*, 89 no. 1(2006): 53–61.

Levin, B. E. "The Obesity Epidemic: Metabolic Imprinting on Genetically Susceptible Neural Circuits." *Obes Res* 8, no. 4 (2000): 342–347.

Levine, A. S., C. M. Kotz, and B. A. Gosnell. "Sugars and Fats: The Neurobiology of Preference." *J Nutr* 133, no. 3 (2003): 831S–834S.

Miles, M. P., & P.M. Clarkson. "Exercise-Induced Muscle Pain, Soreness, and Cramps." *The Journal of Sports Medicine and Physical Fitness* 34(1994): 203-216.

Mustillo, S., C. Worthman, A. Erkanli, G. Keeler, A. Angold, and E. J. Costello. "Obesity and Psychiatric Disorder: Developmental Trajectories." *Pediatrics* 111, no. 4 Pt 1 (2003): 851–859.

Neumark-Sztainer, D., P. J. Hannan, M. Story, J. Croll, and C. Perry. "Family Meal Patterns: Associations with Sociodemographic Characteristics and Improved Dietary Intake among Adolescents." *J Am Diet Assoc* 103, no. 3 (2003): 317–322.

Neumark-Sztainer, D., M. Wall, J. Guo, M. Story, J. Haines, et al. "Obesity, Disordered Eating, and Eating Disorders in a Longitudinal Study of Adolescents: How Do Dieters Fare 5 Years Later?" *J Am Diet Assoc* 106 (2006) 523-5.

Peters, J. C., H. R. Wyatt, W. T. Donahoo, and J. O. Hill. "From Instinct to Intellect: The Challenge of Maintaining Healthy Weight in the Modern World." *Obes Rev* 3, no. 2 (2002): 69–74.

Pinaquy, S., H. Chabrol, C. Simon, J. P. Louvet, and P. Barbe. "Emotional Eating, Alexithymia, and Binge-Eating Disorder in Obese Women." *Obes Res* 11, no. 2 (2003): 195–201.

Raymond, N. C., B. Neumeyer, C. S. Warren, S. S. Lee, and C. B. Peterson. "Energy Intake Patterns in Obese Women with Binge Eating Disorder." *Obes Res* 11, no. 7 (2003): 869–879.

Stein, R. I., L.H. Epstein, H.A. Raynor, C.K. Kilanowski, & R.A. Paluch. "The Influence of Parenting Change on Pediatric Weight Control." *Obesity Research* 13 (2005): 1749–1755.

Strauss, R. S., and J. Knight. "Influence of the Home Environment on the Development of Obesity in Children." *Pediatrics* 103, no. 6 (1999): e85.

Visser, M. "Gregory Bateson on Deutero-Learning and Double Bind: A Brief Conceptual History." *J of the Hist of the Beh Sci* 39 3 (2003): 269–278.

Wang, G. J., N. D. Volkow, F. Telang, M. Jayne, J. Ma, et al. "Exposure to Appetitive Food Stimuli Markedly Activates the Human Brain." *Neuroimage* 21, no. 4 (2004): 1790–1797.

Index

About BOKsystems

BOKsystems is dedicated to health, preventative medicine, and keeping the public up-to-date on cutting-edge research. Initially formed in Houston, Texas, with inspired faculty members from colleges and universities, Body of Knowledge, Inc. has continued to attract enthusiastic experts from other institutions in the United States and abroad. Its mission to promote healthy lifestyles is clear, and people are listening. Government programs and private corporations are offering more funds than ever before to find viable solutions to combat the rise in obesity and related health problems.

While BOKsystems has been in development for a decade, only recently has its founder, Dr. Moore, expanded his vision of the program to reach a larger audience. Over the last few years, he has fine-tuned its focus toward weight management, corporate wellness, and preventative medicine and now this Body of Knowledge concept has been broadened to create symbiotic relationships with other reputable health oriented organizations. But the most important relationship will always be with his patients, members, and subscribers. With prudent alterations to the program in response to public feedback and ongoing research, Dr. Moore will continue to develop the best possible solutions for those who struggle with weight management and health issues.

The Dr. Moore "Story"

After graduating high school in Vacaville, California, Dr. Moore was accepted to U.C. Davis to play football and join his family lineage of engineers. Two years later Dr. Moore transferred to U.C. Berkeley to follow his passion for the biological sciences and graduated with a degree in physiology. There were many employment opportunities on campus, but he found working as a personal trainer was as easy as it was instinctive and continued training clients while attending medical school in San Francisco.

Dr. Moore then moved to Houston, Texas, to complete his residency in foot and ankle surgery. When he started his private practice, he immediately noticed that a large proportion of his patients had weight problems and associated diseases like diabetes, osteoarthritis, and peripheral vascular disease. Then in 1998 he started writing Body of Knowledge and holding classes after clinic hours to discuss weight management with select patients. Frustrated with the prevalence of obesity-related illnesses and the present health care crisis, Dr. Moore then created the Body of Knowledge system.

The decision to build a web site in 2004 combined with the demand for a patient accountability model and preventative medicine system to handle this crisis has recently made his dream a reality. Now with three office locations and still active as a surgical instructor, he continues to work with members of the business and science communities to help more people help themselves.

Dr. Moore is a proud father of twin girls and remains active in Houston with both adult and childhood wellness organizations. He and his daughters enjoy cooking together, biking, water skiing, and other activities that coincide with their Body of Knowledge lifestyle. Dr. Moore plans to keep his focus on childhood obesity, but stay involved with research, and produce more effective programs for schools, employers, physicians, and individual families.